MIASMAS AND DISEASE

MIASMAS AND DISEASE

Public Health and the Environment
in the pre-industrial Age

CARLO M. CIPOLLA

Translated by Elizabeth Potter

YALE UNIVERSITY PRESS
NEW HAVEN AND LONDON 1992

Set in 11/13 pt Baskerville by SX Composing Ltd, Essex, England,
and printed and bound by The Bath Press, Avon.

Library of Congress Cataloging-in-Publication Data

Cipolla, Carlo M.
    [Miasmi ed umori. English]
    Miasmas and Disease : public health and the
environment in the pre-industrial Age / Carlo M. Cipolla :
translated by Elizabeth Potter.
    p. cm.
    Translation of: Miasmi ed umori.
    Includes bibliographical references and index.
    ISBN 0-300-04806-8
    1. Public health – Italy – Florence (Provence) – History – 17th century.
I. Title.
    [DNLM: 1. Environmental Health – history – Italy. 2. History of
Medicine, 17th Century – Italy. 3. Public Health – history – Italy.
4. Sanitation – history – Italy. WA 11 G18 C5m]
    RA508.F57C5813   1992
    614.4'245'51 – dc20
    DNLM/DLC
    for Library of Congress
    91-30385
    CIP

Contents

Introduction

The bulk of this book is not by me. The authors were the physicians, surgeons and magistrates of the Florence Health Board and the Governors of the communities with whom the magistrates corresponded during the first half of the seventeenth century. I should explain. The Florence Health Board, which had been established on a permanent basis in 1527, had its heyday during the first three decades of the seventeenth century. While searching through the surviving documents from this office – documents which are still preserved at the State Archive in Florence – I found a number of reports on the environmental and health conditions which prevailed in the hamlets, villages and towns of the Florentine state during that period. These accurately observed and highly informative reports, written in early seventeenth-century Tuscan, throw a great deal of light on the daily life of a world that historiography has left in the shadows. In bringing these documents into the light I have tried to restrict my interventions and to let the actors in the drama speak in their own spare, effective language; to stand aside as far as possible and allow these actors to come into direct contact with the modern reader. I see my role as that of intermediary, watching closely but rarely intervening.

I did this not only in order to paint a vivid picture but also to give the reader the opportunity of studying directly the way of thinking, theoretical paradigms and semiotic and diagnostic criteria employed by the doctors of that time. (As an aid to understanding, a brief glossary of the most frequently used and linguistically intractable technical terms found in the texts reproduced here will be found at the end of the book.)

The decision to reproduce large portions of the medical reports in their original form has undoubted merits from the scientific point of view. However, this decision may have negative consequences for the general reader who has no particular interest in the history of medicine, in outdated medical concepts or in the medical language of the period. Indeed, it is hard to imagine hundreds of readers poring over the texts presented here, enthralled by what are the often very repetitive accounts by seventeenth-century doctors of events which were sad, unpleasant and often tragic. At the very least the unwary reader will find himself prey to intolerable tedium. I feel it my duty to suggest a remedy. The texts in question are all in Chapter 3. My advice is this: if, after having read a few pages of the medical reports and acquired an idea of their nature and structure, the reader should fall prey to feelings of tedium or depression, he should not hesitate to skip the rest of the chapter and turn to the beginning of Chapter 4 on p. 66. Chapter 4 and the conclusion that follows summarise and comment on the texts of the reports in what I hope is a fruitful and interesting way.

To understand why, regardless of the possible negative consequences, I decided to reproduce these epidemiological reports so fully, it should be remembered that, even today, in order to find out about the pathologies affecting the population of Italy one must refer to statistics on mortality. But as has been pointed out, these statistics can 'at most point up fatality rates but certainly not levels of morbidity'. Figures obtained in this way are therefore very approximate. Further indirect measures of morbidity can be obtained from records of hospital admissions and discharges, from notifiable diseases and finally from general practitioners' medical certificates.[1] The seventeenth-century reports reproduced and analysed here are the result of an intelligent attempt at understanding and are a type of documentation which, although flawed by the deficiencies of the medical science of the time, are lacking in most modern societies.

Nowadays we call infectious a disease caused by parasites such as bacteria, protozoa or fungi. An infectious disease may or may not be contagious. An infectious disease may be transmitted from animal to man (in the case of the plague from rats to man) or from one person to another by means of a vector which could be the flea (in the case of the plague), the louse (typhus), or the mosquito (malaria). An infectious disease is contagious when it is passed directly from one human being to another without the mediation of insect vectors. Syphilis, pneumonic plague and influenza are all examples of contagious diseases. The doctors of the seventeenth century, who knew nothing about the existence and role of microbes and viruses and did not even suspect the part played by vectors, but were firmly convinced of the existence of miasmas and their accursed sticky atoms, spoke generically of 'contagiousness'. In the text which follows this term often appears between inverted commas to show that it is being used in the way in which seventeenth-century doctors used it.

The term *Castello*, which appears frequently in the texts reproduced below, cannot easily be translated into English since it refers to a typically Tuscan phenomenon. A *Castello* was a settlement of respectable size which, being walled, was more than a village, but which, because it was not the seat of a bishop, was less than a city.

Chapter 1

The Health Boards in Italy and Epidemiological Concepts

I have shown elsewhere how between 1348 and 1700 the states of northern and central Italy created the most advanced system of public health and hygiene in Europe with the establishment of health boards, or rather health magistracies, in the major cities.[1] These developments had their origins in the recurring plague epidemics which, starting with the pandemic of 1348–51, devastated different parts of Europe repeatedly and at various intervals. In 1348, right in the middle of that first pandemic, boards were set up in Venice and Florence to deal with the myriad problems created by the catastrophe. The boards set up between 1348 and 1351 and those created during subsequent epidemics were temporary in the sense that the board remained in existence solely for the duration of the epidemic, after which it was dissolved. However, these boards were later transformed into permanent magistracies, in the first half of the fifteenth century in Milan, in 1486 in Venice and in 1527 in Florence. The reason for the change is well illustrated by the Florentine document which established the local health board on a permanent basis in 1527. This document states that it was not possible to 'deal adequately with' the problems created by the epidemic 'without a board which concerns itself specifically with them'; and that furthermore to wait until there was 'the suspicion of contagion' made it 'difficult to carry out that office'.[2]

The transformation of the health boards from temporary into permanent institutions was not a purely bureaucratic administrative process: on the contrary, it reflected the critical shift from a stage of simple, primitive, stopgap measures to a far more mature and intelligent policy of preventive action. It involved not so much the creation of permanent posts and the employment of personnel on a permanent basis as an extension of the area of intervention and a change in the type and quality of those interventions. At the height of an epidemic the bulk of the energies and resources of the health magistracies was absorbed by the setting up and administration of *lazarettos*, the closure of infected houses, the creation of cemeteries reserved for the burial of plague victims, the recruitment of doctors, the organisation of the work of gravediggers. Between epidemics, on the other hand, the permanent health magistracies devoted more attention and greater resources to a whole range of much wider and more varied measures. In the course of time these preventive measures became increasingly numerous and diverse. Thus the health magistracies came to concern themselves with the quality of food on sale; the movements of beggars and prostitutes; the sanitary conditions which prevailed in the houses of poorer people; chemists' shops and the medicines they sold; sewers; the workings of the hospitals; the activities of the medical profession; the sanitary conditions in inns and taverns; the movements of goods, travellers, pilgrims and ships; the quarantining of ships, travellers and suspect merchandise; the issuing of health passes for travellers and goods; the keeping of registers of mortality showing the name, address and profession of the deceased and the presumed cause of death together with the medical certificate, and a hundred and one other things besides.[3]

The ultimate aim of all this intense, even feverish activity which, I repeat, was typical of the northern and central Italian cities and was not found to anything like the same extent north of the Alps or south of Florence,[4] was to prevent and combat the plague. Occasionally the authorities concerned themselves with other diseases such as typhus, malaria, smallpox and influenza; but plague was and remained the principal enemy. Even when cases of smallpox or petechial typhus were discovered, the main worry was that these diseases might develop into a plague epidemic.

This terror of the plague was not unfounded. The pathogenic agent which causes the plague is a bacillus known to microbiologists as *Yersinia pestis* (after its discoverer), which is a normal parasite of rats but not of man. In the course of evolution that *modus vivendi* of greater or lesser reciprocal tolerance which normally tends to be established between a parasite and its habitual host has not developed between man and the bacillus. When *Yersinia pestis* is transmitted to man by means of fleas, the former has no adequate natural defences. In the case of bubonic plague, 70–80 per cent of those infected died within 4–7 days. Plague epidemics were therefore a disaster. In the towns between 25 and 40 per cent of the population normally died within a few months. In the countryside the occasional village might escape the epidemic but in those villages affected by the plague the mortality rate was as devastating as in the towns.[5] Great writers, from Boccaccio to Manzoni and Camus, have used their literary talents to great effect in describing the climate of horror, fear and terror which seized hold of individuals and communities in the face of this disease, but however effective they may be, these literary descriptions nevertheless remain inadequate.

As we have noted, plague is caused in man by a bacillus known as *Yersinia pestis*, which is a habitual parasite of rats and some other rodents such as squirrels and marmots. The disease is transmitted to man by fleas (usually *Xenopsilla cheopis*, the rat flea) which become infected by sucking a sick rat's blood and then, when the opportunity arises, transmit the bacillus to man. In these, the classical cases, the sequence of transmission of the disease is rat → flea (*Xenopsilla cheopis*) → man. However, research carried out by French epidemiologists and microbiologists in North Africa, as well as what can be inferred from medieval documents, suggests that the human flea (*Pulex Irritans*), although much less dangerous than *Xenopsilla cheopis*, may act as a vector, compensating by its numbers for its intrinsic inefficiency as a vector. This would give the sequence man → flea (*Pulex irritans*) → man. Finally there is the case of those individuals affected by plague who develop secondary pneumonia and spread the disease through the expectoration of particles of bacillus-laden mucus (droplet infection). In such cases, which are rather rare but absolutely deadly with a fatality rate approaching 100 per cent, the sequence is a direct one, man → man.

It is evident from the above that in the absence of rats and fleas there is no risk of plague. But if rats and fleas are abundant, there is every chance that an epizootic disease will be transformed into an epidemic. At the time, however, no one knew this. The paradigm of medical science consisted not of microbes and their vectors but of humours and miasmas. As far as plague was concerned, people spoke of an ill-defined but universally recognised 'corruption and infection of the air', which degenerated into highly poisonous 'sticky' miasmas that killed the person they infected, either by inhalation or by contact. According to the theories of the time, the 'corruption and infection of the air' could be caused by an inauspicious conjunction of the stars, vapours rising from marshy water, the eruption of volcanoes, foul and filthy conditions or exhalations arising from 'rebus et corporibus putridis et corruptis'.

The miasmal atoms could be absorbed through inhalation or skin contact. Skin contact could be direct but could also take place through the handling of objects to which these poisonous atoms had 'stuck'. Some believed that the miasmatic atoms could be transmitted to man by contact with certain animals, particularly furry ones such as cats and dogs. According to the theories of the time, the sequences of transmission could be: miasma → man; infected object → man; infected animal → man; man (infected) → man. The circuits of infection imagined by contemporary theory were therefore simpler but more numerous than those identified by modern science. Hence the frenzied zeal with which health officials of the period set to burning clothes and furniture which they believed to be infected, disinfecting merchandise and correspondence and placing ships, goods and people under quarantine.

The history of medicine in Europe from the end of the classical age to the beginning of the modern era is the curious story of a

fundamentally mistaken theoretical paradigm which nevertheless succeeded in dominating and conditioning medical thought
for an exceptionally long period of time. How and why a totally
erroneous paradigm maintained for centuries its uncontested
domination of the field of medical science has been and remains
one of the most fascinating problems in European cultural
history. Part of the explanation lies in the elegant simplicity,
rigorous logic and internal consistency of the theoretical model.
There was no lack of men endowed with great intelligence, indis-
putable rationality and acute observational abilities among the
doctors of Europe between the thirteenth and eighteenth centuries. And yet not even men of high intellectual calibre ever
dared to question the humoral-miasmatic paradigm whose
clarity, logic and consistency were sanctioned by antiquity and
tradition. Time after time correct factual observations were
made and recorded but, by some perverse mechanism, what was
correctly observed did not cast doubt on the validity of the prevailing paradigm but was dialectically adapted to that very
paradigm to serve as further proof. For example, doctors soon
observed correctly that plague epidemics normally broke out
during the hot summer months. It never entered their heads that
this might be in some way connected with the proliferation of insects such as fleas. It was during the hot summer months that
people's senses were most violently assaulted by the nauseating
smells of manure, excrement and filth which choked the hamlets,
villages, towns and even cities of the time. The recurrence of
plague epidemics during the summer months therefore paradoxically served to confirm the time-honoured sequence of dirt →
smells → miasma → pestilence. To give another example: doctors were quick to notice that those who dealt with furs, carpets,
bales of wool and cloth were more likely to contract plague than
those who dealt with marble, iron or wood. The idea that the
furs, carpets and bales of wool might harbour infected fleas did
not even cross the doctors' minds; the theoretical paradigm did
not leave any room for microbes and their vectors. The doctors
saw in the correctly observed facts proof that the atoms of
poisonous miasmas, being 'sticky', obviously stuck or adhered
more easily to hairy surfaces than to smooth ones.

Today with hindsight it may seem strange that no one thought to blame rats and fleas, but we must remember that rats and fleas were a constant presence in the society of the time. Since there were rats and fleas in abundance at times when there was no sign of plague, it was not illogical to exonerate them from all responsibility when the plague suddenly and unexpectedly appeared.

Thus the story of medical thought in those centuries is a classical example of the truth that the correct gathering of objective facts is not in itself sufficient to lead to valid conclusions. 'Facts' are like the tiles of a mosaic; on their own they mean nothing. What is needed is a theory which brings them together in a meaningful whole. And the theory must be correct; if it is mistaken it may serve to distort the meaning of the facts. On the other hand, theories do not come from nowhere; they are derived from the observation of facts. It is therefore a question of continual feedback between the formulation of theoretical hypotheses, verification by means of observation of the facts and experimentation, and reformulation of the theory on the basis of experimentation. The story of medical thought between the twelfth and seventeenth centuries shows that paradoxically it is much easier for people to adapt the observed facts dialectically to the ruling paradigm than to renounce the ruling paradigm in response to possible new interpretations of the facts.

Accounts in English of the history of medicine and epidemiology give great prominence to the public health movement founded in Britain in the nineteenth century during the age of cholera by men of the calibre of Benjamin Disraeli, Sir John Simon, Dr William Farr and Sir Edwin Chadwick. The courageous and praiseworthy work of these and others who joined them is regularly and justifiably extolled and the people in question are described as brilliant innovators and pioneers of a new era. It is a great pity that in the course of this glorification no mention is ever made of the fact that what was done in England in the nineteenth century was nothing more than an almost identical repetition of what had previously been done in Northern Italy between the fifteenth and seventeenth centuries. I do not make this point for reasons of vulgar national pride: the clarification is important because it shows how the paradigm which dominated medical science and epidemiological practice remained substantially unchanged from the Middle Ages to the last quarter of the nineteenth century. John Simon, William Farr and Edwin Chadwick acted in ways and according to paradigms which were still those which had informed and guided the actions of Italian health officers in the fifteenth, sixteenth and seventeenth centuries.

At the time of Sir Edwin Chadwick's *Report on the Sanitary Conditions of the Labouring Population* (1842) the prevailing theory in the best medical circles was still that of miasmas.[6] Chadwick and his collaborators acted and behaved not only as if all 'smell' was disease but also as if all disease was 'smell'.[7] Chadwick's chief recommendations in his Report and during the years following 1842 were: (a) the compulsory removal of all rubbish; (b) the improvement of the sewerage system; (c) street cleaning.[8] We shall see later that these were also the major concerns of the Italian health officers of the fifteenth, sixteenth and seventeenth centuries.

In the course of these brief remarks it will have become clear how and why dirt and smells occupied a position of primary importance in the concerns of Italian health officials at the end of the Middle Ages and the beginning of the modern era.

As has been shown by Alain Corbain in his book *Le miasme et la jonquille*[9] and by Piero Camporesi in his scholarly introduction to the Italian edition of the book,[10] filth, smells and rottenness pervaded every corner of Europe. Even in periods when there was no epidemic, therefore, the Magistrates for Health were never free of worry, tormented as they were by the terror that the dirt and smells which besieged them might corrupt the air and explode in a plague epidemic. On the other hand, given the lack of medico-pathological knowledge, the frequent, widespread influenza epidemics, cases of malarial fever and intestinal infections could not fail to raise fearful spectres and feed the terror that when such illnesses reached a certain level of intensity they might be transformed into a plague epidemic. Hence the various inquiries, so modern in spirit,[11] which the Florentine Health

Magistrates carried out into the sanitary conditions in various parts of the state during the first half of the seventeenth century.

The documentation regarding these inquiries can be divided into two broad categories. One group consists of the replies sent by local authorities (usually the representatives of the central power such as Podestà, Capitani or Vicari) in response to specific requests for information on the sanitary situation, requests which were normally sent by the Florentine Magistracy when it received news of an increase in mortality. This first category can be divided into two further groups. There are inquiries carried out by the Magistracy into a single locality and there are those which involved several localities or even whole regions. To this second subgroup belongs the general inquiry of 1622, which will be dealt with in the next chapter.

The second group of documents consists of the inquiries carried out directly by the Magistracy by sending experts to the place concerned. Following their inspection the experts were required to present a written report to the Magistracy. This second group of inquiries can also be subdivided. There are reports by technicians (engineers, master masons, master roadmen), which are concerned mainly with the technical problems of sewerage, drains and graveyards; and there are medical reports written by doctors sent on missions by order of the Florentine Magistracy from the places where they practised their profession to the places about which the Magistracy wanted precise and impartial information.

In a typical health inspection a doctor who had been requested to visit one or more places would arrive in the appointed place and make contact with those locals who were able to provide him with the information necessary to assess the situation. Thus he would contact the community doctor (if there was one),[12] with whom he would discuss recent cases of sickness and death. He would contact the priest and examine with him the parish registers in order to assess the course of mortality and try to obtain from him information about the causes of death. Finally, if there was a pharmacy the Health Board's envoy would also consult the pharmacist to obtain information about the availability of medicines. More often than not the envoy would then visit some of the sick. He also had the task of giving advice and instructions to the local doctor and authorities about the treatments to use and sanitary measures to adopt in the battle with the disease. After this the envoy would go on to the next place he had to inspect or would go home and write the report which was to be sent to the Florentine Magistracy as soon as possible.

Chapter 2

'Miasmas, Filth and Rubbish'

On 14 July 1622 the Florentine Health Magistracy sent the following communication to the Grand Duke: 'Since our Magistracy has been informed that in many parts of the State the inhabitants are up to their necks in filth, as the saying goes, in order to ward off all disorders in such dangerous times, we sent a general printed letter to all governors on 4th May last ordering that all filth and rubbish be taken out of the cities, villages and *castelli* of the dominion; and that the greatest possible cleanliness should be maintained inside the houses; and that if there are full cesspits they should be emptied; and that every other thing which might cause harm by its smell should be seen to; and that care should be taken around sewers and stagnant water which are not covered over in order that they should not damage health by foul vapours . . . and that they should send one of their notaries to visit and make sure everything was done correctly, with orders to take note of everything which it might be necessary to do and immediately inform the Magistracy of this.'[1]

Orders to keep every village 'clean and free from every sort of nasty thing' had already been given in 1607–8. In May-June 1621 the keeping of trays of silkworms, which were extremely smelly, was prohibited in Empoli, Borgo S. Sepolcro, Pistoia, Volterra, Livorno, Castelfiorentino, San Miniato, Pescia,

Arezzo, Scarperia, Cortona, Pietrasanta, Lucignano and Pisa.[2] On being informed that in many places people were 'up to their necks' in filth, and fearful of the consequences such a situation might have on general sanitary conditions, above all 'at such a dangerous time' when Italy and Florence itself were in the throes of a typhus epidemic,[3] the Florentine Health Magistrates returned decisively to the problem of filth; and on 4 May 1622 they sent the ordinance mentioned in the letter to the Grand Duke to the 'cities, lands and *castelli* of the dominion'. (The text of the ordinance is reproduced in full in the Appendix to this book.)

The ordinance required the local authorities to have one of the administration's notaries (1) collect precise, firsthand information on the sanitary conditions of the territories under their respective jurisdictions; (2) send the information collected immediately to the Florentine Magistracy; (3) publish the text of the order requiring private citizens to eliminate dirt and rubbish from inhabited areas; and (4) ensure that the order for a general clean-up was observed.

Table 1 lists the communities which received the ordinance and whose reply to the Florentine Magistracy survives. The ordinance was also sent to other communities whose reply, however, has been lost. For those communities for which documents survive, Table 1 gives the date on which the order was received by the community, the date on which it was published and the date on which the information requested was sent to Florence. A comparison of the dates will show that at least as regards points (1), (2) and (3) the communities acted with considerable speed. As for point (2), the reply of the Podestà of Bibbiena gives an effective and telling description of the ways in which the ordinance was published: the Podestà writes that the order was published 'to the sound of trumpets in the most frequented areas so that everyone might know about it and copies were affixed to the columns'.[4]

In 1622 the Grand-Duchy's administration completed a census of the population of Florence and the Florentine state.[5] The Florentine Health Magistracy's inquiry of the same year provides us with a census, so to speak, of the 'filth and rubbish'.

TABLE 1. *Chronology of the circulation of the order of 4 May 1622*
and the replies of the local authorities

	Date of receipt of ordinance	Date of publication of ordinance	Date of local authorities' reply to Magistracy
Buccine	8/5	8/5	9/5
Figline	7/5	7/5	10/5
Castiglion Fiorentino			11/5
Bibbiena		13/5	13/5
Montelupo		8/5	12/5
Fucecchio	7/5	8/5	12/5
Borgo S. Sepolcro		14/5	16/5
Montepulciano		14/5	16/5
Castelfiorentino	12/5	14/5	17/5
Castelfranco di sotto	12/5	15/5	17/5
San Gimignano		18/5	18/5
Volterra			19/5
Modigliana		12/5	20/5
Cortona		10/5	20/5
Empoli		12/5	20/5
Pratovecchio		15/5	22/5
Campiglia			22/5
Pontedera			24/5
Fiorenzuola		16/5	24/5
Bagno	13/5	15/5	25/5
Montecatini			25/5
Cutigliano		15/5	29/5
Pisa			31/5
Pieve Santo Stefano	11/5	11/5	31/5
Marradi	9/5	9/5	1/6
Borgo San Lorenzo	9/5	9/5	1/6
Certaldo	18/5		4/6
Anghiari			8/6
Vicopisano		15/5	10/6
Bientina e Buti		16/5	10/6
S. Giovanni, Montemagno, Cap.		17/5	10/6
Noce, Cunigliano		18/5	10/6
Arezzo		14/5	10/6
Montaione	20/5		10/6
Buggiano	14/5	20/5	14/6
Greve	24/5		16/6
Pescia	16/6	18/6	26/6

Note: The first number indicates the day; the second indicates the month.

TABLE 2. *Description of the inhabitants of the city of Florence and contado [surrounding countryside] and of the whole of the Florentine dominion made in 1622.*

City of Florence within the walls	76023
Florentine contado	
VICARIATE OF S. GIOVANNI	2368
Montegonzi	2126
Montevarchi	5360
Bucine	4381
Laterina	1270
Terranuova	4427
Loro	1616
Castelfranco	3723
Figline	3962
Greve	5653
Pontassieve	10773
Reggello	7269
	52928
VICARIATE OF CERTALDO	2870
Poggibonsi	2532
Castelfiorentino	2850
Montespertoli	4285
Radda	6418
Gambassi	2744
S. Casciano	5919
Barberino	4812
Montelupo	4911
Lastra	980
Empoli	7078
Galluzzo	29072
	74471
VICARIATE OF SCARPERIA	6740
Dicomano	1984
S. Godenzo	1119
Borgo S. Lorenzo	6532
Vicchio	4888
Barberino	5019
Carmignano	3889
Campi	10884
Fiesole e Sesto	10796
	52051 (51851)
VICARIATE OF S. MINIATO	3397
Castelfranco	5805
Fucecchio	4558
S. Croce	1834
Vinci e Cerreto	3215
Cigoli	2681
	21490
Town of Pisa and contado	
Town of Pisa	15461

Lari	2829
Peccioli	7256
Palaia	5653
Rosignano	738
Vico Pisano (Bientina)	5949
Cascina	5587
Pontedera	4274
Librafatta (Ripafratta)	4248
Livorno	*12413
Pietrasanta	11034
Fivizzano	10737
Castiglione del Terziere	6827
	92992

Town of Livorno ('settled' i.e. resident population)	2000

Town, contado and mountain areas of Pistoia

Town of Pistoia	8386
Cortine di Pistoia	16002
Serravalle	9201
Tizzana	4153
Montale	6792
Montagna di Pistoia	9277
Terra di Prato e suo contado	16786
Pescia	7142
Buggiano	8692
Montecatini	4759
Vellano	2641
Montecarlo	4234
Barga	5540
	103605

Town of Volterra and Colle and its Capitanato

Town of Volterra	8679
Colle	4911
S. Gimignano	4725
Sasso, Leccia, Lutignano	636
Montecatini e Gello	973
Pomarancie	2070
Querceto e Sassa	463
Monteverdi e Canneto	490
Castelnuovo di Val di Cecina	870
Montecastelli	617
Bibbona	1281
Campiglia	816
	26531

Town of Arezzo and Val di Chiana

Town of Arezzo	8286
Cortine di Arezzo	10110
Civitella	3556
Cortona	15371
Castiglione	6391
Lucignano	2964
Foiano	4131

Marciano	1009
Montepulciano	6432
Valiano	394
Anghiari	3627
Monterchi	1798
Subbiano	1827
Borgo S. Sepolcro	6943
	72839

Casentino

Poppi	3425
Montemignaio e Battifolle	1809
Ortignano	1073
Pratovecchio	2999
S. Lorino del Coante	1567
Romena	1705
Castel S. Niccolò	3244
Bibbiena	2425
Castel Focognano	3704
Pieve S. Stefano	2680
Chiusi	1296
Caprese	1793
Badia Tedalda	2409
Verghereto	2511
Sasso di Simone	2209
	34849

Romagna

Terra del Sole	2338
Modigliana	3995
Rocca S. Casciano	1852
Marradi	3141
Palazzuolo	2938
Geleata	4408
Dovadola	1189
Premilcuore, Montalto e Corniolo	2597
Portico	991
Sorbano	701
Bagno	5473
Tredozio	1721
Firenzuola	7773
	39117

---

* Biblioteca Nazionale di Firenze, Magliabechi, II, 1, 240. The totals given here are those given in the original document. Totals obtained from the sum of partial figures are given in brackets.

Professor L. Del Panta, who kindly pointed this document out to me, has also brought to my attention the existence of a 'Summary of the souls in the old State of S.A. made in 1622', which is kept in the Archivio di Stato in Florence, Miscellanea Medicea f. 229 ins. 2 (fascicolo 12). In this second document the population of the Florentine state is sub-divided into different administrative districts from those used in the list reproduced above. As regards the population totals there are some discrepancies between the two documents but in general the data agree well.

The picture which emerges of the living conditions in one of the most advanced areas in seventeenth-century Europe is simply horrifying.

One of the most conspicuous sources of the appalling smells, and a continual danger to public health, was the inadequate sewerage system; and indeed, in some cases, the total lack of sewers and cesspits. In his report of September 1607 the master mason Lucini wrote that Castelfranco was pervaded by the 'stench emanating from certain places where sewage runs which are open and lack cesspits' and that 'they must empty the cesspits that exist because they stink'. In Santa Croce 'some pools and cesspits stink and in one place where the rainwater and waste water cannot escape they putrefy'. In Bientina 'things are very badly arranged because the [chamber] pots, all inadequately set just below the commodes, let the waste run out through gaps in the walls and fall into certain narrow alleys between the houses in which [the inhabitants] throw all the dirt and rubbish from their houses. The result is that so much stuff accumulates in these alleys that even when it rains the rainwater is not sufficient to carry it out to the ditches designed for that purpose; and the small proportion which does come out gets stuck in certain ditches next to the walls. The result is a stench and filth so awful that it is quite impossible to live there.'[6] Five years later the situation in Bientina had not improved. Gherardo Mechini, who was sent there on an inspection in June 1612 with Dr Barziono from Pisa, found that 'None of the houses has a privy with its own underground cesspit but they shit between the houses where there are gaps between the walls and where the water from the roofs should carry the stuff away, but this does not happen because the place is not on a slope . . . and there are hundreds of turds to be removed which, as well as stinking horribly, present an extremely disgusting sight to those who pass by in the street. And there are many houses in this place whose privies empty into certain horrible backyards and open courtyards which look and smell so disgusting that this alone would be enough to bring on the plague when it is very hot.'[7] At Vico in 1610 an envoy of the Florentine Magistracy found that 'this place is scarcely less filthy than Bientina having neither privies nor sewers and they tell me that in the heat of summer they can hardly bear to walk down the streets for the stink'.[8]

On 8 October 1622 the Podestà wrote from Bibbiena that 'in this place there is an alley about 40 braccia [24 metres] long into which run several sewers from open cesspits [belonging to twelve families] who for the most part do not have privies in their houses. These families throw their waste out of the windows, so that all the time there is a lot of waste matter and filth, which continually gives off such a stink and stench that it troubles the neighbours and could easily cause many serious diseases, especially through the corruption of the air.'[9]

In July 1609 the Podestà of Fucecchio had complained that in the town 'there is a narrow alley which, although it is covered above and on one side, is used by the inhabitants who live on either side to throw all their waste into; and to tell the whole truth [they use it] as a cesspit as well, which makes a terrible stink and stench so that if you walk down the main road next to it you have to hold your nose.'[10] Little more than a month later the same Podestà was writing to the Magistrates as follows: 'there are 63 [houses] which have uncovered cesspits which give off an unbearable stench at this time of year.'[11] On receiving the Magistracy's order of 4 May 1622 the Podestà of Fucecchio set one of his officials the task of making a more precise assessment of the hygienic and sanitary conditions of the place. On 12 May the Podestà wrote to Florence that the envoy had brought back horrifying news: 'he told me with great amazement . . . that he found that all the privies drain out of the houses in the open and all this excrement is gathered together, which stinks terribly and is disgusting to see; because even if you go along the street you can see all the filth. Of the 350 or 400 households in this place there are very few which have a cesspit in the house as they have in other places.'[12]

In reply to the ordinance of 4 May 1622 the Capitano of Marradi wrote on 1 June that 'there are some cesspits along the river which runs through this *castello* into which everything falls from above and stays there on the dry bed until the river carries it away; so that if the river doesn't rise the stuff isn't washed away'.[13] On 17 May the Podestà of Castelfranco wrote that 'of all the places in this area of jurisdiction there is not one which is filthier than this *castello* and the reason for this is that between the rows of houses there is a narrow alley into which all the cesspits empty and the filth from the alley runs into the street and stinks greatly'. Convinced of the absolute necessity of undertaking the construction of some sort of sewerage system, the Podestà concluded his letter with the hope that 'an expert be sent to see and give instructions because there is no one here with that kind of expertise'.[14] The Magistracy responded to his request by sending a master mason, Cosimo di Andrea Mazantini, to Castelfranco. In June of that year he confirmed that 'inside the *castello* all the privies enter into certain alleyways about two braccia [120 centimetres] wide between the rows of houses, and the privies of all the houses lack drainpipes so that the waste falls in the open and runs on to the main streets and stinks terribly. In order to remedy this filthiness it is necessary to build a vault under the main street and to build a cesspit underground which should be four braccia [about 2.4 metres] deep; and all the houses which have privies should build covered drainpipes; and everyone should pay their part of the cost.' Mazantini reckoned the cost of the work at 360 scudi.[15]

From Montopoli master mason Mazantini reported that 'as for the open privies inside the *castello* they are in a terrible state; and in my opinion all those listed below [there follow the names of twenty persons including the poor hospital and the priest's house] should all build cesspits and drainpipes with their own outlets'.[16] In 1622 the Vicario wrote from Castel S. Giovanni that 'there are four or five alleys into which all the households throw their waste; and they have no sewers, which makes this *castello* stink'.[17]

Animal excrement was added to that of man. In the first place there were the horses, asses and mules used for transport, which were kept in stables attached to the houses inside the villages. This was not a particularly serious problem. Those who could afford to buy and keep a horse, ass or mule could usually afford to pay a servant to clean the stable. The animals had their 'straw bed', and dung would occasionally accumulate there: but the whole thing normally remained within tolerable limits. Problems arose above all when the dung removed from the stables was not taken to the fields but was left in a heap, for example on the road around the walls. Thus in September 1607 master mason Lorenzo Lucini reported that in Bientina 'they keep the manure from their stables outside on the road next to the walls, where it rots and stinks terribly'.[18] However, apart from horses, asses and mules many villages contained large numbers of other animals which created far more serious problems.

On 7 October 1607 the administrators of the community of Castel S. Giovanni wrote to the Florentine Magistracy that 'the statutes of Castel S. Giovanni permit each family to keep a pig for fattening within the *castello* and this year there is a huge number of these animals. Since in our opinion they stink horribly and since there is an unseasonably large number of sick people here, we pray your Lordships to empower the Vicario to order all pigs to be removed from the *castello* within four days . . . and this for a certain period, departing just this once from the statute and not including those which the butcher keeps for slaughter.'[19] In May 1610 the administrators of Portico di Romagna informed the Magistracy that 'they have a statute forbidding the keeping of pigs and since the penalty is small and ignored by transgressors and governors alike, therefore no notice at all is taken of it. And this is how a large number of pigs comes to be kept in the *castello* at the moment and the stench from them is so bad that one can hardly bear to walk along the streets; and there is also a risk that the filth will cause an infection of the air.'[20] In September 1607 Lorenzo Lucini wrote that in Santa Maria a Monte 'some reduction must be made in the number of pigs, since nearly every household has one and their sties stink to high heaven'.[21]

At Pontedera there was 'no order or statute prohibiting the keeping of filth and rubbish in the *castello* or around the walls'. However, there was a provision in the statutes on the basis of which 'the butcher may keep as many animals as the citizens of the Commune of Pontedera agree to'. In May 1613 the Podestà wrote that 'in this *castello* it would be very beneficial to the health of the people if the butcher were forbidden to keep any kind of animals inside the *castello* because they stink'.[22]

In November 1613 it was reported from the *castello* of Laterina that 'there are many pigs, some raised by the inhabitants and others owned in partnership by people from outside, and these [pigs] are the cause of much dirt in the streets, squares, loggia and even in the courtroom, and there is a great risk that the air will be infected and human bodies corrupted since the streets of this place are narrow and always full of rubbish and the pigs root around and cause an unimaginable stench'. In Laterina there were statutory regulations which decreed that 'no one in the said *castello* may keep or cause to be kept more than two pigs and a breeding sow' and 'that no pig may wander about the *castello* without supervision' but the statutes were disregarded and 'there are families who keep eight or ten of them'.[23]

Regarding the *castello* of Pontedera, in December 1613 the Florentine Magistracy received 'sure and certain information that a large number of pigs, lambs and sheep raised by the inhabitants are kept in the *castello* and therefore one sees great quantities of filth, which cause a terrible stench; and the said inhabitants have the habit of throwing excrement, urine and other filth out of the windows and they keep heaps of muck, manure and other filth in the *castello* itself; and just as it must be suspected that these were the cause of the diseases which have afflicted this place in the past, so it may be believed that in the future they may have a very bad effect on public health.'[24]

In Lorenzo Lucini's report of 1607 mentioned above we read that in Vico Pisano 'there is a great stink caused by the large number of geese which they keep there. This should be remedied by keeping fewer of them and enclosing them in poultry houses.'[25] In June 1622 the master mason Cosimo di Andrea Mazantini, who was responsible for carrying out an inspection in the Val d'Arno, wrote that 'several herds of sheep are permitted to stray in the *castello* of Fucecchio and this must be stopped and they must be kept out of the *castello* because they smell horribly and make a lot of mess'.[26] In July 1628 the priest of Palaia informed the Magistracy that 'the butcher of Palaia, Pollonio di Nicolò Boscagli, keeps forty to fifty sheep and two pigs in a room at the end of the main street which was fully occupied by houses on either side. At present it is impossible to stand at the doors or windows because of the stench.'[27]

The agriculture of the time suffered from a serious shortage of fertilisers which regularly created a bottleneck in agricultural production. The principal fertiliser was manure, or to put it bluntly, animal excrement. But there was never enough manure, so that peasants who farmed land in the vicinity of the towns would regularly buy cartloads of stinking human waste from those whose job it was to empty the cesspits. What the peasants wanted, however, was the 'solid stuff' (also known as 'stuff for peasants'), which was considered 'good for manure', and not the 'soft stuff' (also known as 'watery stuff'), that is, the liquid which was no good as fertiliser.[28] In view of the prevailing scarcity, the peasants of the time devoted a great deal of time to the collection and storage of manure, which was for them a raw material of primary importance. The consequences of these practices in terms of hygiene and fragrance did not, however, commend themselves to those who were not peasants. In 1607 in Ponte di Sacco, master mason Lucini noted that 'around the main road everyone has a piece of land and puts the manure there to rot, where it festers and makes an unbearable smell'.[29] In August 1610 the nuns of the convent of Santa Giustina in Santa Croce complained that 'within the walls [of the village] near the convent people have made a ditch where they get their manured waste for their [the peasants'] own benefit without showing any respect for this holy place, where we are prevented by the stench from celebrating the holy offices in church'.[30] Again in Santa Croce in 1627, 'towards Grasciano there are ditches, or rather charcoal pits, which belong to the community: in some parts of these there is stagnant water and in these same charcoal pits there are several pits full of manure put there by various people to rot down and then be taken to their fields for the current sowing'.[31] In May 1622 around Fucecchio 'piles of manure' could be seen (and smelt) 'around the *castello* and along the main street'.[32] Still in May 1622 in Castelfranco, 'people are still keeping many piles of manure, which stink greatly, outside the walls'.[33] In the *castello* of Santa Maria in Monte 'there are many open huts full of

manure outside which give off a great stench'.[34] A certain Gherardo Mechini, accompanied by Dr Barrione from Pisa, was sent
by the Florentine Magistracy to Bientina in June 1612 to carry
out an inspection. These two reported that they found 'the place
in an appalling state and both the streets and squares so disgusting and so full of waste that the stalls of animals are less
filthy. And there is even manure in the streets and squares piled
up against the houses, which the people leave there to rot; this is
not only disgusting, it also stinks to high heaven.'[35]

   The most pathetically tragic aspect of this business, however,
was that of the people, whose poverty was so abject that they collected the manure they found in the streets and took it home
where they kept it until they had accumulated a sufficient quantity to sell. In July 1628 the Provveditore of Castelfiorentino sent
the Florentine Magistracy 'a note of those who keep heaps of
manure at home and these people do not keep animals but collect it [the manure] in the street and take it to their houses'. The
nine people listed in the 'note' included three widows, two other
women, 'the messenger of the place who is extremely poor' and
three others.[36] According to an officer of the Magistracy who
visited Castelfiorentino in 1627, these poor wretches who collected dung in the streets in order to sell it 'earn enough from this
to pay their rent'.[37]

To the problems of human and animal waste and the collection,
storage and composting of manure was added that of stagnant
water. Bientina in 1610 'was surrounded by a ditch called the
Cilecchio ditch into which water drains from the marsh; and
because it does not run freely during the summer it gives off a
great stench, especially because the people put the linen there to
steep'.[38] In May 1622 in Castelfranco 'around the walls outside
the *castello* are some vegetable gardens which are surrounded not
by a hedge but by a ditch where there is a lot of stagnant water
which stinks; in some places the water is two or three braccia
[1.5–2 metres] deep and since it is so low down and the land is
flat it is hard to drain it'.[39] In Pontedera 'there are some ditches
around the *castello* in which the water stagnates and in hot
weather it putrefies and sends dreadful smells into the *castello*,

whose walls have been demolished, and this could cause great
harm . . . in some places the ditches have been breached to take
earth for making bricks'.[40] In Castelfranco di sotto 'there were
two reservoirs which have been abandoned and the only water
that goes into them is what passes through the street and comes
out of the manure heaps and it putrefies in such a way that it
could cause the plague; and they use this water for washing and
for extinguishing lime mortar and they keep it for fear of the fire
spreading because the clean water is a quarter of a mile away'.[41]

Environmental sanitary conditions were further damaged by a
variety of productive activities whose by-products or waste pro-
ducts were harmful, or at the very least offensively smelly. Particular mention should be made here of the cultivation of silkworms, the retting of linen and hemp and of butchery. In
Bientina in 1607 'in the main street there is a pit underneath the
butcher's shop from which rotten matter overflowed and ran
down the street making a stench'.[42] In Montopoli, again in 1607,
the butcher had 'a gully inside his house which is full of all kinds
of filth, excrement, guts and other muck, which make the most
cruel stench, together with a heap below the shop entrance on to
which all the bloody waste falls, giving off an unbearable
stench'.[43] In Figline in 1618 'in many places there are many
heaps of manure and other rubbish which can make the air fetid
and in addition great quantities of rubbish have been dumped
and continue to be dumped around the gates; and in particular
butchers dump stuff there every day'.[44]

The Podestà wrote from Castelfiorentino in 1627 that 'in this
place there are two slaughterhouses both within the *castello*, in
which a great number of animals are butchered, which cannot
help but create a stench; and it would therefore improve matters
a great deal to order the building of a slaughterhouse for the
slaughter of these animals along the River Elsa so the guts and
blood could be thrown into the river'.[45]

The butchers, with the stink of their bloody and rotting waste,
were not the only ones to corrupt the air. In Volterra in 1615 the
rope-maker Bastiano Ciangherotti of Empoli, 'leaving aside the
smelly nature of the trade itself [because of the steeping of the

hemp], practises it in such a way that his shop where he makes
the rope stinks so much that his neighbours in the street of Santo
Agnolo, one of the main streets of the town and one in which
many nobles live, suffer greatly'.[46] In Castelfiorentino in May
1622 'Agostino Ticciati has opened a tannery in his house, the
stink of which is very damaging to his neighbours'.[47]

In Tuscany the locating of cemeteries away from inhabited areas
was made compulsory by a series of ordinances dated 2 January
and 11 March 1777, 25 April 1780, 2 September 1783 and 19 and
28 April 1784. Before these dates the practice prevailed of 'carrying the corpses to the burial places uncovered and displaying
them in the churches and burying them there'.[48] It happened
particularly during periods of higher than usual mortality that
the graves inside the churches were not made as they should be:
the holes were not deep enough and the tombs were not properly
sealed. In September 1607 master mason Lorenzo Lucini was
sent from Florence to inspect a vast area of the Florentine state
and he found that graves presented a serious problem. In Fucecchio six graves in the Church of S. Salvadore 'smelt a bit', six-
teen graves in the cloakroom of the Compagnia della Beata Ver-
gine 'smelt' and eighteen graves in the cloakroom of the
Compagnia di San Giovanni 'smelt a lot'. In Castelfranco 'they
do not take proper care [of the corpses] and so they stink'. At
Santa Maria a Monte 'I found three hastily buried corpses
which smelt because the hole was not deep enough and they
were not properly covered'. At Peccioli, Lucini called a mason
'because of the smell of corruption in the church' and had him
'close up all the graves in the presence of the Podestà and
myself'. At Marti 'the church smelt somewhat when I arrived; I
called in a mason and had [the tombs] sealed with lime mortar
and the same thing with two others which were under a portico
at the top of the cemetery and smelt a bit'. At Montopoli 'there
are seventeen graves in the Compagnia della Croce next to the
church and they give off an unbearable stench. With great difficulty I found a mason and with even greater difficulty a bit of
lime mortar.'[49]

Bad smells are unpleasant and represented a form of pollution.

In this particular case, however, it was not merely a question of unpleasant olfactory sensations: there was also the absolute conviction that bad smells could, from one moment to the next, provoke an epidemic of the dreaded plague. It is not surprising, therefore, that the health authorities were set on waging war on dirt and smells. To this end they did not hesitate to take drastic and even extraordinary decisions. Writing about Bientina in his report of 1607, Lucini the master mason concluded: 'in addition to working on these smells and stenches it would be of great benefit to the health of the *castello* to break down [the walls] at the end of certain streets because only the middle street is open at both ends; the others are all dead ends where the winds cannot blow and clean them out, so all kinds of stench accumulate and remain there.'[50] Despite the drastic nature of the proposal the Florentine Magistracy did not wait for it to be repeated, but had the walls of Bientina demolished to aerate the town. In August 1611 the Cancelliere of Pontedera wrote: 'I went to Bientina and from what I could learn I discovered that in the previous year, in the interest of health, Messer Gherardo Mechini, His Most Serene Highness's engineer, had ordered the walls to be demolished so that the wind could pass in and out.'[51]

The Magistracy's actions did encounter opposition, caused by ignorance, lack of will, vested interests, habit, poverty or a misguided spirit of independence. On 3 June 1622 the Podestà of Bibbiena wrote that he had ordered all manure to be removed from the town: 'discovering that some people had not obeyed I ordered them to remove the manure which is in public places, otherwise I would have it removed at their expense. Nevertheless, they have not obeyed.'[52] On the 27th of the same month the Podestà of Barberino del Mugello wrote: 'In this town there is a square next to the Podestà's Palace and in this square there is a church, and there is a space between the said palace and the said church about eighty braccia [48 metres] wide; and on Saturdays a large number of cattle are gathered there and deposit so much dung that it is impossible to leave the house. The said space slopes towards the palace and when it rains all that filth runs down towards the palace. And there is a well in front of the said palace and the said filth spoils the water in the said well and the place is so horrible that it is impossible to live there. I protested and last Saturday I made them go down to the river where they used to go; and some of them said they wanted to see who was the cuckold who ordered them to go away and they made them come back just to spite me.'[53] On 4 September 1624 the Podestà of Castelfiorentino wrote: 'I have given orders through my envoy that no one may keep pigs or sheep in the stables of Castelfiorentino in order to remove all the smells and stenches which could cause disease, and furthermore gave them written notice; nevertheless they refused to obey me and mocked at my orders.'[54] The Podestà of Castelfranco di sotto wrote in May 1622 that 'until now there has been little obedience, partly because of the great poverty and partly because they don't take much notice until someone has been put in prison'.[55] In June 1622 Cosimo di Andrea Mazantini reported from Fucecchio that 'as for the heaps of manure the Potestà published the order and no one wanted to obey. It is therefore necessary that Your Lordships make them an order with penalties and punish someone otherwise these smells will not be got rid of.'[56] Commissario (Commissioner) Guiducci, who was sent to Castelfiorentino in October 1627 to give the Podestà a hand in a difficult public health situation (see p.63) wrote that: 'These people are unruly and since they have not been punished for disobeying orders in the past they will always continue to do so, so that it would be a good idea to make an example of someone in order that great clemency should not give rise to contempt.'[57]

Owing to the Magistracy's efforts in some communities the sanitary conditions showed some improvement; but in many others things continued as before.[58] Until very recently filth and rubbish dominated the European scene.

Chapter 3

Medical Reports and the Florentine Health Magistrates

As we saw in chapter one, the Florentine Health Magistracy frequently received precise information, or just heard rumours, to the effect that morbidity and mortality levels in a certain area of the state were higher than usual. During the first four decades of the seventeenth century, if this happened the Magistrates usually investigated the situation for fear above all that the problems might be a sign of the imminent outbreak of a plague epidemic. As has already been mentioned, these investigations by the Magistracy could take one of two forms: (a) the Magistrates could limit themselves to a request for written information, a request which was sent to the local representatives of the central Grand-Ducal authority (that is, the Podestà, the Vicario or the Capitano) or the local doctor (if there was one); or (b) they could despatch to the area a doctor of good repute, normally from a neighbouring district, who would assess the situation after consultation with the local doctor (if there was one) and the parish priest; and, having consulted the parish death register and visited a few of the sick, would write a report which he sent to the Magistracy. While he was in the area the Florentine Magistracy's envoy also had the task of collaborating with the doctor and the local authorities in taking the necessary measures for appropriate care of the sick and the control of the epidemic.

In the Archivio di Stato di Firenze I traced ten or so substantial medical reports, together with a certain number of less important reports and brief occasional reports written between 1608 and 1627.

The doctors who were sent on inspections were always physicians with a university doctorate. Some of them were destined for brilliant careers. For example, Antonio Durazzini, who was the community doctor in Borgo S. Sepolcro in 1622 and in that year was sent on an inspection tour to San Vito, Figline, Castel S. Giovanni, Montevarchi and Borgo S. Sepolcro, reappears in 1630 as a member of the powerful College of Physicians in Florence.[1] Cesare Ruschi, who was a doctor in Santa Maria in Monte in 1611–12 and, as we shall see, was sent on an inspection of Campiglia in 1611, turns up again in 1630 practising in Pisa, the city of his birth, where he became among other things physician to the local bishop.[2] More will be said about Latanzio Magiotti, who was community doctor in Borgo San Giovanni and later became physician to the Grand-Ducal court (see p. 57). Others spent their lives in rural areas, moving sometimes from one small town to another for family or financial reasons.[3]

The doctors often refer in their reports to the number of deaths they have derived from the parish registers. For Fucecchio in 1608 Dr Pucci reported that 'from the middle of July to the middle of August there were thirty or so deaths among children, old people and others' (see p. 32). For Bibbona in 1615 Dr Collodi reported that 'between January and now [8 May] about sixty people have died, both adults and children' (p. 52). However, things were not always so clear. In his inspection in 1610 of Marciana, Cascina, Pontedera, Peccioli, Ponte Sacco, San Pietro in Colle, Bientina and Vico Pisano, Dr Bagnone reports only the number of adult deaths. We suspect of this limitation from the fact that the list of deaths supplied by the doctor did not contain anyone under the age of fifteen. This suspicion becomes a certainty when the figures supplied by the doctor are compared with those obtained from a surviving parish register. For Vico, which he visited on 26 March 1610, Dr Bagnone reported that 'In January a 25-year-old man died with a pustule on his chest, in February a 50-year-old woman died with a pustule on her thigh, in March an old man of eighty died suddenly.' However, the parish register for Vico Pisano has the following figures for the period 1 January – 26 March 1610:[4]

1610,	3 January:	a son of Niccolaio di Riccio
	6 January:	a son of a policeman
	9 January:	Giulio di Antonio di Vico
	22 January:	a daughter of Cosimo di Ninsa
	8 [sic] Jan:	a son of Filippo di Salvadore
	5 March:	Menchino the goatherd
	?	Giovanna sister of Brugiaferro
	12 March:	a son of Michele Battaglia

Similarly, in his report written in Pisa on 29 April 1610, Dr Cartegni wrote that 'in this month [April] twelve people died [in Vico]'. However, the Vico parish register records thirteen adult deaths and four children.[5] The discrepancy between the thirteen deaths on the register and the twelve recorded by Dr Cartegni can be explained by the fact that the thirteenth death occurred on 29 April when Dr Cartegni had already left Vico and was in Pisa, from where he sent his report to the Magistracy. The information in the register therefore confirms that Dr Cartegni too excluded 'children' from the death tally. The explanation for this practice lies in the fact that even in normal times children and young people died in such high and fluctuating numbers that there was no sense in including them when assessing the gravity of the epidemiological situation. Furthermore in Florence too the civic death rolls did not include the deaths of children or adolescents.[6]

The members of the Magistracy were not doctors. Given the state of medical knowledge at the time, an average level of general culture was more than sufficient to permit the interpretation and evaluation of the reports. However, when the Magistrates received the reports they made use of the assistance of doctors who were employed in Florence and directly dependent on the Magistracy (cf. for example p. 61).

The remainder of this chapter consists of the essential portions of the reports presented in chronological order. The following chapter contains some reflections suggested by the reports in the

wider context of the medical, social and economic history of
those centuries.

Summer 1608   The Florentine Magistracy learned of several cases
of sickness occurring in the area of Fucecchio, Castelfranco di
sotto, Santa Maria in Monte and San Miniato and instructed Dr
Ludovico Pucci, born in Montepulciano but practising in San
Miniato,[7] to visit these places and assess the health situation. 'In
accordance with these orders', Dr Pucci began his inspection in
August in Fucecchio. As soon as he arrived in the little town
Pucci contacted Aluigi Guidoni da Palaia, the community doctor. Dr Guidoni was convalescing from 'fevers brought on by
overwork' but this did not prevent the two doctors from having
'a long discussion about the diseases prevailing in that place
[Fucecchio] and the surrounding area'. Dr Guidoni reported
that 'in the surrounding countryside there are many sick people
who do not seek treatment but live in a very disorderly manner
so that in his opinion as many die for that reason as die from
malignant diseases. He said that these illnesses began with tertian and double tertian fevers with *accidenti* occurring on the
seventh or eighth day, namely extraordinary thirst and some
delirium, and these brought death without the appearance of
petechiae.'

Dr Guidoni added that petechiae had appeared on four
patients but 'since the relatives and helpers of [these four people]
were around them, and indeed slept in the same bed and room,
without however falling ill', it must be concluded 'that the sickness came from the wicked intemperance and bad way of life of
those who fell ill rather than from contagion'.

'As for the people of Fucecchio,' Dr Guidoni reported, '[the
disease] could very well have the same cause because they are all
labourers who return home exhausted and live in a disorderly
way, and since they are full of bad humours they fall ill with
similar fevers and he affirms that many died rather because they
do not look after themselves than because of contagion or the
malignity of the disease.'

After his interview with the local doctor, Pucci visited various
sick people and came to the 'same conclusion' as Dr Guidoni,

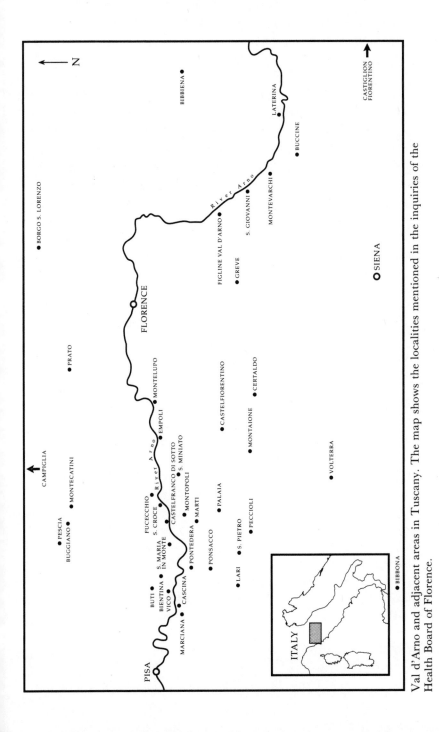

Val d'Arno and adjacent areas in Tuscany. The map shows the localities mentioned in the inquiries of the Health Board of Florence.

adding that 'although some of them had treatment they died from the great quantity and evil quality of humours, as often happens in every kind of place'.

Before falling ill, Dr Guidoni had about 80 patients in his care, 30 to 35 of whom were purged while others had blood let 'and they did not want any other treatment'. According to Dr Guidoni, more patients had survived than died.

However, Dr Pucci wanted to find out whether the number of sick in the areas had increased or not while Dr Guidoni was ill. He therefore sent 'the messenger of the Podestà around the houses and he found that the number [of sick] is 191 but most of them have not called the doctor, either because they are too poor or because they have little faith in medicine'.

As well as Dr Guidoni, the community doctor, there was a young doctor in the town, Dr Valerio Galleni da Fucecchio. Dr Pucci went to see him too. He learned that Dr Galleni had 'some patients with tertian and double tertian fevers and that about the seventh [day] they suffer from malignities with an increase of fever, blackened tongue, very great thirst, restlessness and loss of appetite but there are no petechiae and [some] recover from these *accidenti* while [others] die'. Dr Pucci, who seems to have been a conscientious man, decided to visit 'many' of these patients with tertian fever and concluded that 'what he [Dr Galleni] said seems to be true'.

Going on to visit the parish priest, Dr Pucci learned that '30 or so people, children, old people and others, died between the middle of July and the middle of August'.

Before leaving Fucecchio Dr Pucci also inspected the pharmacy. His impression was 'that as far as the quality of the medicines, by which I mean the electuaries, is concerned, they could have been better, but they are not so bad that they cannot be used; and as for the quantity there would be sufficient for very many people if they would purge themselves and have faith in medicine. And since the chemist is a man who has the means, if he sold them he could send to Florence every day for fresh supplies. So there would be no problem with the medicines or their quantity if the majority of people would undergo treatment.'

Dr Pucci 'could not discover the precise number' of sick in the surrounding countryside 'but there are many of them and the rumour is that they are as many [as in Fucecchio]'.

From Fucecchio Dr Pucci went to Santa Maria in Monte. Here 'there is no doctor or chemist' so that 'in order to have information about the prevailing illnesses' the doctor met 'the representatives and other men of the place and in particular the very reverend Ipolito Ristori, who is the canon and parish priest of the place, all of whom told me that there were large numbers of sick': about 50 in the town and about 300 in the surrounding area. The first thing Dr Pucci asked was 'whether the fevers came every day or on alternate days'. From what his informants told him and visits he made to the sick 'just to be sure', the doctor concluded that 'they are tertian and double tertian fevers and not contagious diseases because [those who] frequent and spend time in the same houses do not experience any contagion'.

In Santa Maria in Monte Dr Pucci found that only 'few undergo treatment [for the illness] because of poverty or because of the scant faith in medicine as is typical of this place: however, they do not die, except that twelve have died in the past fifteen days'.

When in a place such as Santa Maria in Monte there was neither a resident doctor, nor a surgeon, nor a chemist (normally both a sign and a consequence of the place's poverty). It was usual for a doctor to come every so often for a day from a neighbouring community and examine those who wished to make use of his services. Dr Del Dua visited Santa Maria in Monte twice a week from Montopoli (p. 45). Often the community doctor of Castelfranco, Messer Flaminio Bernardini, would be 'called in'. When Dr Pucci visited Castelfranco he conferred with Dr Bernardini and asked him for information on the health of the inhabitants of Santa Maria in Monte. 'He stated that the prevailing sicknesses in Sant Maria in Monte are tertian and double tertian fevers, which at first do not appear serious but in some cases petechiae appear on the fourth or seventh [day].'

In Castelfranco and its territory Dr Pucci found a similar situation to that in Santa Maria in Monte, that is tertian and double tertian fevers. In the town he counted about 50 sick and reckoned about the same number for the countryside, 'and from

June until now six or seven people have died'. 'As for the chemist in Castelfranco, apart from bezoar stone, which he says he has sent to Florence for, he has remedies, syrups and waters suitable for such sicknesses and in good quantity.'

The instructions given to Dr Pucci by the Florentine Magistracy did not specify a visit to Santa Croce. 'Nevertheless, since I was passing,' the doctor who, as we have seen, was a conscientious man, decided to ask ' some people about the numbers of sick. They replied that between the village and surrounding country there were about 100 sick, who were not dying of the sickness.'

Dr Pucci practised in San Miniato al Tedesco. In his report he wrote of this place that between 8 June and 15 August 'of those I treated none died except a friar of San Domenico of acute fever in seven days'. Note the restriction, 'of those I treated'. In fact there was more than one death in San Miniato. In an accompanying letter dated 15 August 1608 sent with Dr Pucci's report to the Florentine authorities, the Grand-Ducal Vicario wrote that 'as for deaths, I have learned from priests and others that in the past twenty days ten or twelve people have died in San Miniato although the doctor says only one died; and indeed three people died today'.[8] The Vicario explained this discrepancy between the doctor's figure and his own by observing that 'it may be that he [the doctor] does not know [the number of deaths] because he may well not have treated those people'. In fact, many people did not consult the doctor because of poverty, but the suspicion remains that Dr Pucci underestimated the number of deaths not from ignorance but in order to put his own activities as community doctor in a good light.

As for the sick, Dr Pucci reported that 'in the town there are at most thirty people sick with tertian, double tertian and continual tertian fevers, of whom only one woman developed petechiae but then recovered, although some among the thirty are dangerously, but not desperately, ill. As for the countryside, I hear that there are many but I cannot say how many because the peasants treat themselves and hardly ever consult the doctor, either because they are too poor to pay for the treatment or because they have little faith in medicine, as is usual among country people.'[9]

1610   The Florentine Magistracy was informed of abnormal levels of morbidity in the area of Marciana, Castello di Cascina, Pontedera and Ponte di Sacco. On 18 March it noted that 'some traces remain of the sickness which swept Pontedera, Cascina and Ponte di Sacco and other surrounding areas two years ago', so the suspicion was that the same sickness had re-emerged. The Magistrates were alarmed not only by news that 'many people were falling sick and a considerable number dying' among the civilian population but 'by the number of soldiers who have died month by month and continue to die according to the lists sent by the Cancelliere of that band'. Mindful of 'the dangers and problems encountered the other time the sickness occurred in these places through not having provided the necessary remedies promptly', the Magistrates decided to send urgently 'a medical expert to visit those places which are affected and gather full information about the disease, its cause and effects and give a detailed account of it all' to the Magistracy. Given the proximity of Pisa to the affected area, it was decided to send a doctor from Pisa, 'which would be cheaper'.[10] The choice fell on Dr Giovan Battista Cartegni da Bagnone.

Giovan Battista Cartegni da Bagnone matriculated at Pisa University in November 1582 and graduated in medicine in October 1587.[11] In the 1620s Dr Cartegni was reader in 'Theory of ordinary medicine' at the University of Pisa and in 1628 he published a short *Treatise on the Winds as they pertain to the Medicine and Location of the City of Pisa*.

Dr Cartegni carried out his inspection in three days during March 1610. According to his report, 'the prevailing sicknesses in this area are catarrhs of thick and viscous phlegm which descend from the head to the throat creating anginas [commonly called *shiranzie*] and in some cases this substance is so abundant that it suffocates them, stopping their breathing. In some cases it descends from the throat to the chest and fills the lungs and the lung cavity, causing great difficulty in breathing, called asthma by doctors, and great stertor or wheezing can be heard and some have tightness of the chest and abundance of these humours and are weak; so being unable to expel this humour they are suffocated; others, in whom the quantity is less and who are robust and broad-chested, manage to expectorate it, but with difficulty and over a long period. In some cases there can be found pleurisies, known as pain of the ribs [pain in the side], and peripneumonias, that is inflammations of the lungs.'[12]

According to Dr Cartegni the winter had been 'cold beyond measure and snowy'. During the cold weather the heads [of the peasants] had become filled with humours. These humours should have fallen 'from the head to the throat' but this did not happen during the winter months and Dr Cartegni explains this by the assertion that owing to the intense cold the phlegmatic humours were 'frozen and unable to move' and for that reason had remained blocked in people's heads. The first warm days of spring 'made these humours mobile by liquefying them and opening the passages, which happened at the end of winter; at which time the sun being near the equinox gives out a good deal of warmth, especially on those who stay out uncovered in it [the sun] as these peasants normally do who are always out in the sun'. In addition, according to Dr Cartegni, in the latter part of the winter there was 'snow and cold which were felt particularly at night and had the effect of squeezing the humours which had already been made runny by the daytime warmth of the sun and making them fall to the throat and chest'.[13] This ingenious but absurd and amusing explanation was not the product of Dr Cartegni's fruitful imagination: as will be seen, other doctors gave the same explanation, with minor variants.[14]

Dr Cartegni's report is dated from Pontedera on 22 March 1610. Evidently worried about the state of public health, the Florentine Magistracy decided not to wait for Dr Cartegni's report before undertaking another inquiry and sending to the area 'one of the principal doctors of this city [Pisa], Dr Bagnone', accompanied by 'a surgeon so that if it should be necessary to carry out any autopsies in order to understand better the causes of these sicknesses it may easily be done'.[15]

Dr Bagnone arrived in Marciana on the evening of Saturday 20 March 1610. 'I went to this place first,' he later wrote in his report, 'because I had been told some days earlier in Pisa that there were many sick people there and that some had died in a very short space of time. I immediately found the parish priest and asked him how many had died in February and March and with what symptoms, and he showed me the book where these things are written down.' The doctor noted that, excluding children, four people aged between 35 and 62 had died in the two months, all from 'descent of catarrh from the head to the throat and chest'.[16] Having consulted in the parish death register, Dr Bagnone wanted to see the situation for himself. 'In order to understand what had happened,' he wrote in his report, 'I went round the town and found that the majority had suffered from or continued to suffer from this sickness, either badly or less badly; and they had survived rather because of strong constitutions than because of medicine because they do not undergo any treatment.' In connection with this he related that: 'Among these [patients] there was one who was in desperate straits. A pilgrim chanced to stop there and had them boil together in water barley, honey and bran, and with this he made a poultice and put it round the patient's neck. This caused the tremor to stop and he spat up a lot of stuff and cleared it; and this remedy was not without sense and shows that if the patients would accept treatment more would recover.' In a final note the doctor reported that 'in some other cases the catarrh has descended to the legs and made them swell a great deal. There were no petechiae or malignant fevers. This is what the parish priest, a diligent man, informed me and I have not seen any sign of them.' From Marciana Dr Bagnone went to the *castello* of Cascina on Sunday, 21 March. In Cascina he immediately contacted the parish priest and had him show 'the book where he keeps account of deaths'. The book showed that in the months of February and March four adults had died: one woman died of pleurisy, the others had been ill for some time but the immediate cause was 'the descent of catarrh to the chest'.[17]

Mastro Giulio, 'an old and experienced surgeon', lived and practised in Cascina. Dr Bagnone sent for him and asked if there were sick people in the place. The old surgeon replied that 'there were only four or five' and took the doctor to see them.[18] Notice that when the visiting doctor wanted to meet with a local colleague, he paid the latter a visit. In the case of the surgeon, on the contrary, he was summoned to the doctor's quarters. This difference in behaviour can be explained by the rules of etiquette. The surgeon, regarded as a manual worker, belonged to a class which was distinctly inferior to that of the medical doctors.

Having visited the sick of Cascina Dr Bagnone asked mastro Giulio, 'who rides around here every day if had seen petechiae or other signs of malignity and he told me he had not, but only sickness of the kind described above'. On Monday, 22 March Dr Bagnone was at Pontedera. The community doctor was an old acquaintance of Dr Bagnone, who thus did not feel obliged to call on his colleague as the rules of etiquette demanded but sent for him in a friendly and familiar way, asking him to come and see him. The local doctor, together with the parish priest, reported that six adults had died in Pontedera in February and March: one 'with inflammation of the lungs and catarrh on the chest', one with 'suffocating catarrh', a third of pleurisy, two more of 'catarrh in the throat and chest'.[19] 'And two recovered from these illnesses.' As for the numbers of sick, Dr Bagnone noted that at the time of his visit to Pontedera there weren't any, 'only a few have light catarrh and are not in bed'. He asked the local doctor 'whether he had come across any malignant illnesses and petechiae and he told me he had not seen a single one this winter'.

On Tuesday, 23 March Dr Bagnone was in Peccioli. He immediately conferred with the curate and the local community doctor, from whom he learned that nine adults had died in February and March, six of them of 'catarrh on the chest', one of 'inflammation of the chest', one of dropsy and one of postnatal infection.[20] Three other people had fallen ill but recovered. On the day of his visit there were no sick people in Peccioli except 'a woman with an ordinary fever', and Dr Bagnone does not seem to have visited her. In addition, Dr Bagnone noted that according to Peccioli's community doctor 'in the places nearby, that is Terricciola, Bagno ad acqua, Soianezza, Soiana, Morone, Casa nuova there are four sick in all, one with pleurisy and three with fever and catarrh. And he has not seen any petechiae nor other signs of malignant fever.'

Dr Bagnone learned from the doctor of Peccioli that the village of Orciatico near Volterra had been 'badly hit by these sicknesses which are going around'. Wanting more recent and fuller news the doctor mingled with people in the market. The doctor's words bring this typical scene from the pre-industrial world to life: 'So in order to find out more I had the market in Peccioli searched to see if there was anyone there from that place [Orciatico]; and two were found who told me that in less than two months up to that day more than thirty adults had died; and on asking them the symptoms of the sickness I found that, as the doctor had also told me, they were the same as those described above. They said that many of the sick had pains in their shoulders and in various parts of the body, others had swollen throats, and with all of them the catarrh eventually went to their chests and they died within nine days at most, but most in less than that, in three, four or seven days.'[21]

March 24th   Dr Bagnone was in Ponte Sacco, where the usual procedure was repeated. The doctor contacted the parish priest and consulted the parish register of the dead. He found that in the months of February and March thirteen adults with ages ranging between 15 and 55 years had died. Four had died after 'long illnesses': the other nine suffocated by 'catarrh on the chest'.[22] 'Of these [dead] very few had any treatment' was the comment.

Dr Bagnone obtained information about 'the nature of the sickness' of those who died 'from the parish priest who had visited them several times and from the surgeon of the place'. The priest and the surgeon informed him that 'there were no petechiae or other signs of malignity: and none of them suffered from angina'. On the day of the inspection there were only two sick people in Ponte Sacco whom Dr Bagnone examined, giving a diagnosis of pleurisy for a 35-year-old and 'catarrh on the chest with very severe infection' for a girl of 14. On the same day, 24 March, Dr Bagnone visited S. Pietro in Collina near Peccioli. He learned from the curate that seven adults had died in February and March.[23] 'The priest informed me,' he writes, 'of the symptoms of the sickness which are the same as the others, that is catarrh, some cases of pleurisy, and some inflammations of the

lungs. They have not had inflammations of the throat but great
pains in their ears, others have had pain in all their limbs. And
as well as those who died [the priest] says that most [of the inha-
bitants] of this place have had pains in the ears and many of
them had great quantities of horrible discharge from their ears.
No petechiae or other bad signs have been seen. Now only one
person is suffering from this sickness.'

On 25 March Dr Bagnone arrived in Bientina. There were no
doctors in the town: three of them had died 'in a short space of
time'. Dr Bagnone obtained the information he required 'from
the parish priest who keeps an account of deaths in a book and
on the nature of the illness', and from the chemist. He learned
that during the months of February and March seventeen adults
had died in the *castello*, nearly all of them of the usual catarrhs
and pneumonia.[24] 'Very few' had sought treatment. Still on the
basis of what his informants said, Dr Bagnone reported that 'no
petechiae or other bad signs were seen'. There were four sick
people in the *castello* on the day of Dr Bagnone's visit to Bientina.
The doctor examined them and compiled the following list:

M. 57 years, ill for nine days with catarrh on the chest and pains
   but not pneumonia; he spits well and should recover;
M. 60 years, ill for nine days with pains in the head and fever
   caused by catarrh;
F. 48 years, ill for five days with pneumonia and in grave
   danger;
M. 27 years, ill with pains in head and ears and matter on his
   chest.

Dr Bagnone's inspection ended on 26 March with a visit to the
castello of Vico. The doctor met the parish priest, the surgeon and
the chemist and was assured that the town had enjoyed 'good
health all through the winter'. Only three adult deaths had
occurred during the months of February and March.[25] 'Now
there is only one person who is seriously ill and that is Pierino
the innkeeper, who at first had inflammation of the throat and
then the matter descended to his chest and he cannot get rid of it
and will die. He has been treated from the beginning and I

examined him. And there are two women ill with fever but in no danger.' Some inhabitants of the *castello* took the opportunity offered by the doctor's visit to inform him that 'a large part of the cause of the sickness which has afflicted the *castello* has been the great quantities of filth, human and animal, which are found in the street; that all the streets are in disrepair and that they would like some steps to be taken because in the summer the *castello* stinks to high heaven'.[26]

As we have seen, Dr Bagnone concluded his inspection on 26 March. The following day, 27 March 1610, the Magistracy of Pisa wrote with laudable promptness to the one in Florence that 'Dr Bagnone has returned after visiting six more places and written a report on each one, which I send to your Lordships. And when we asked him if he thinks these illnesses will increase with the warm weather he replied that he was rather of the opinion that they were likely to disappear with the warmth.' The question about the likely effects of the seasonal rise in temperature reflected the usual fear that with the arrival of summer the existing epidemic might turn into a plague epidemic. As has been seen, Dr Bagnone dismissed this hypothesis.

The letter also mentioned the payment of Dr Bagnone for his services. With characteristic stinginess the Medicean authorities had made him a payment of 30 *scudi*: 'he was given 30 *scudi* and even though he must have little left over he has not asked for further payment.'[27]

A month later, at the end of April, however, the news reaching the Magistracy from Bientina and Vico was again not good. They again approached Dr Cartegni, who was sent to visit the place once more. On 29 April 1610 Dr Cartegni submitted his second report.[28]

With regard to Bientina, Cartegni wrote that 'in these months many people have died of chest illnesses, that is catarrh, which is so thick and abundant that they cannot spit it up, often being too weak, so that finally it suffocates them; and also some from pneumonia and peripneumonia, that is inflammation of the lungs. And they died in the space of four, seven or nine days.' In the doctor's opinion, 'these illnesses are of the same type' as

those described in his previous report (see p. 36) 'and are not
malignant and are going around in many parts of Italy'. As for
the patients, the doctor noted that 'very few of these people of
Bientina undergo treatment and they lack doctors, for if they
underwent treatment the majority of them would recover. I
found many who are still ill with this sickness but most of them
are not in danger if they undergo treatment as I urged them.'

As for the treatment to be used, Dr Cartegni showed himself to
be a man of good sense, advising against excessive use of phlebotomy: 'it would be good if they were provided with a doctor and
not left to a surgeon and not bled as has been done in the past.'[29]

As far as conditions in the village were concerned (conditions
which as we have already seen were indescribably filthy) Dr
Cartegni wrote: 'As for the quality of the air of Bientina it is of its
nature bad since it is near the lake from which bad vapours rise
continuously. . . . In addition, they have a cause of illness very
close by on their own land and this is their faeces, which they
dispose of in the houses and within the walls very close to the
houses since they do not have privies nor sewers which can carry
such filth and keep it from sight, and the filth is in the open in
many places, the resulting stench being such that I do not know
how it does not bring on the plague.' The conditions of work
were not very favourable either: 'they are almost all fishermen,
in the water all the time, and they always go to the lake at mid-
night, whatever the weather.'

In Vico at the end of March Dr Bagnone had been informed
by the priest, the surgeon and the chemist that the *castello* had
'enjoyed good health all through the winter' (see p. 40). At the
end of April Dr Cartegni found that the situation had deteriorated markedly: 'twelve people died this month and several fell
ill.'[30] And the doctor could not refrain from remarking that 'this
place is scarcely less filthy than Bientina, having neither privies
nor sewers and they tell me that in the summer they can hardly
go into the streets for the stench'.

In Buti Dr Cartegni encountered the widespread belief that
'the rice fields are the source of their ills'. The doctor inveighed
at length against this idea and reaffirmed his belief that 'as for
the illnesses which are going around now, as has been said they

are affecting many parts of Italy, some of which enjoy the purest air, and as they write to me from Lunigiana many have died in Pontremoli and yet it has some of the purest air to be found anywhere'.

An inspection could be an exhausting undertaking because of the problems posed by travel and transport. In April 1611 Dr Cesare Ruschi was sent from Pisa to Campiglia to ascertain the local health situation and give any directives that might be necessary. On the eighteenth of that month the doctor wrote directly to the Grand Duke, informing him that 'I arrived in Campiglia late this evening and am so tired that I am unable to stand and since I arrived here I have been able to speak only to the "Chief of Justice" who told me of the nature of the sicknesses, which in fact have been only *scherantia* [inflammations of the throat] and the epidemic has passed its peak even though as he told me many people are still ill. . . . Tomorrow I shall see the doctor and see and hear everything and give such orders as may be necessary . . . I left Pisa yesterday at eighteen hours and since the coachman did not know this road I had to take a guide, who exhausted me.'[31]

Two days later, on 20 April 1611, Dr Ruschi, having assessed the situation, wrote to the Magistracy giving his conclusions: 'I came to Campiglia to see what sicknesses prevail here and their courses and I find that at present good health reigns, there being only six sick, of whom two are women with pain of the chest, namely stitch, two other cases of double tertian fevers and two girls aged seven who have a slight inflammation of the throat, called *scheraentia*, and whose chances of recovery are good, even though they are so young that they cannot be given the necessary treatment. But there was no sign of any malignity or contagion in these patients, as we had feared from the number of sick and dead which there had been there. But having had an excellent account of the past sicknesses both from the doctor and from others, I learned that of the sixty people who died between the beginning of March and now, twenty or so were children who died of smallpox and the rest, some of pleurisy, some of fever,[32] but the majority from *scherentia* [inflammation of the throat] which developed not only because of the inflammation of the internal muscles of the larynx but because of the great abundance of phlegmatic humours which fell to those parts from the head. And this meant that in two or three days they were suffocated by the quantity of stuff which accumulated in that part of the head.'

The deaths of twenty children from smallpox and about forty adults from infections of the respiratory tract in the space of one month out of a population which did not exceed one thousand were occurrences which one would expect to have produced a livelier reaction on the part of Dr Ruschi.[33] However, the doctor was evidently concerned to reassure the Magistracy that 'the epidemic has passed its peak'. Furthermore, as we shall see in the next chapter, the doctors of the time did not imagine that there could be anything contagious in a long series of deaths caused by 'suffocation by catarrh'. Dr Cartegni's theory on the origin and diffusion of broncho-pulmonary infections has already been quoted (p. 36). Dr Ruschi's theory did not differ substantially from that of Dr Cartegni.

According to Dr Ruschi, 'at the end of the past winter the brains of these people [were] filled with humidity owing to the great quantities of rain or southern winds which prevail in this place, and Hippocrates states clearly: austri auditum habitantes at caput gravantes. Consequently in the spring the slight warmth outside shifted the matter but could not disperse it, because the morning and evening air being still cold blocked the pores. The matter the expulsive virtue of the brain caused it to descend into the throat below it where having become compressed, *scherantia* [inflammation of the throat] to develope and because of the large quantity of matter which accumulated there they suffocated within a short time.'

Dr Ruschi's 'theory' was analogous but not identical to that of Dr Cartegni. While for Cartegni it was the first springtime sun which made the 'phlegmatic humours' which had been frozen in the brain 'runny' and 'opened the passages' making the humours 'descend to the throat and chest', for Ruschi it was the continuing cold which caused an excessive formation of harmful humours and dampness in the brain so that a 'compression' was created, in reaction to which the 'brain's expulsive virtue' pushed 'the matter' down 'to the throat and chest'. In his report Dr Ruschi shows himself to be aware of and sensitive to the socio-economic factors which contributed to the diffusion of the disease. 'We must also consider,' he writes, 'that the majority of those who died were poor peasants exhausted by hard work and inadequately fed, as the poor tend to be.' In addition there had been 'a lack of medical care since most of them are poor and only send for the doctor when they need the priest'.[34]

1612:   The alarm sounded for Santa Maria in Monte. Even judged by the standards of the day, the medical service in the community was inadequate. There was Dr Attilio Del Dua. Born in Montopoli he had matriculated at the University of Pisa in 1590 and graduated in philosophy and medicine in 1595.[35] He does not seem to have been a bad doctor according to the standards of the time but he came to Santa Maria only two days a week, dividing his time between Santa Maria and Montopoli, where he lived and practised. As he himself told the Magistracy in March 1612, 'few if any [of the sick in Santa Maria] have been treated, some because of their poverty, others because [Dr Del Dua] did not get there in time to treat them since he lives in Montopoli, which is three miles from Santa Maria, with an obligation to go there twice a week although in this period he went there every time he was called; but since there is neither a surgeon nor a chemist's in Santa Maria in Monte it was impossible to use those treatments which the sickness requires from the beginning.'[36]

Faced with such a situation the Florentine Magistracy acted swiftly and decisively. It ordered Dr Del Dua 'to go to Santa Maria in Monte and stay there until we see that the sickness takes a turn for the better'.[37] The Magistracy stated that the doctor 'will be paid for his work but if he disobeys [he will be sentenced] to prison since this is an express order of His Most Serene Highness' [the Grand Duke].[38] Furthermore, 'in order that there should be someone to carry out blood-letting [the Magistracy ordered that] an assistant surgeon from the hospital of Santa Maria Nuova [in Florence] should be sent and take with him medicines and remedies both from the pharmacy of the

hospital and from the Grand-Ducal pharmacy, judging it to be
an act of great charity to provide them with remedies and medicines because the majority of them are very poor and we have
been assured by the said Dr Del Dua that many have not been
able to be treated because of their extreme poverty'.[39]

They must have thought in Florence that Dr Del Dua did not
have the necessary knowledge and experience to deal with the
situation, however, and they decided to send a Florentine or
Pisan doctor of good repute to Santa Maria in Monte to carry
out an inspection. It appears that Dr Alessandro Pietramaloschi
was chosen for the task on the personal initiative of the Grand-
Duke. He went to Santa Maria and wrote his report on 21 March
1612. He reported that according to what the inhabitants had
told him 'seventy people have died in two months, almost all
from the *accidenti* of pleurisy and angina; the former was harsh
without sputum and turned into pneumonia or suppurated, then
[the patients] became empyemic and eventually died; while the
latter is not the kind of which Hippocrates spoke in the *Apho-
risms*, which has an external cause, nor yet that kind which he
speaks of in the second book of *Epidemics*, which sort of angina is
caused by the scatica of vertebrae inwards; but it is preceded by
inflammation and of this type he speaks in the third book of the
Prognostics, dividing it into three types; and these poor people
died of each of these, since some had atrocious pain in the throat
without the appearance of any tumour, difficulty in swallowing
and great difficulty in breathing when partly lying down, which
is the certain, inseparable symptom of the first kind of angina
which is most terrible and is called *synanche* by the Greeks, and is
caused by the inflammation of the muscles of the larynx. It may
well be that the inflammation was not pure and uncomplicated
because of the mixture of phlegmatic humours, and these
patients died within a few hours. The other kind called *synanche*
by the Greeks, as Galen clearly distinguishes, originates in the
inflammation of the internal muscles of the throat without great
difficulty in breathing except when a greater quantity of matter
is carried to the larynx; but it causes great difficulty in swallowing, and pain without any apparent tumour as in the first type.
The third and last type is called synanchic effect, where the

throat appears very swollen, and even though this is good both as a sign and as a cause, nevertheless most died of this kind.' The report does not end here but continues for several pages with disquisitions on the winds and their possible influence on the course of the epidemic.[40] As we saw, Dr Pietramaloschi's report is dated 21 March 1612. Did the excess of erudition and the corresponding lack of precise, down-to-earth information on the course of the epidemic not satisfy the Florentine Magistracy? Or was it difficult to keep a well-known Florentine doctor in Santa Maria in Monte for a prolonged period? Or was it perhaps too expensive? We are in the realms of speculation. The fact is that on 26 March the Magistracy indicated that it had ordered Dr Cesare Ruschi, whom it had sent to Campiglia the previous year (p. 43), to go to Santa Maria in Monte, assess the situation and suggest suitable treatments and measures to be taken.[41] Dr Ruschi wrote his report on 29 March: 'On Your Lordships' orders, I came to Santa Maria in Monte to treat these patients; and here I found Dr Attilio Del Dua and we discussed both the present and past sicknesses. And he informed me that the past sicknesses were pleurisy, angina and parotitis and that many had died from them. . . . The current sicknesses are angina, pleurisy and some putrid fevers caused by the putrefaction of bilious and phlegmatic humours which on being transmitted to the throat create anginas, if [transmitted to] the pleura which encloses the ribs [cause] pleurisy. And these illnesses are by their nature extremely acute and fatal especially when combined as they are with malignant fevers, as are those who die on the fourth and seventh day because of the malignity of the wicked humour. But it is commonly believed that they are not contagious diseases but common sicknesses which affect now one place, now another and God forbid they should be contagious as we should all be sick by now; but nevertheless they are serious and refractory diseases and many have died of them.'

Dr Ruschi was well aware that the prevailing morbidity could not be explained solely in medico-biological terms but reflected also particular social and economic conditions. Already in his 1611 report on Campiglia he had pointed out that 'the majority of those who died were poor peasants who were exhausted by hard

work and badly fed, as the poor tend to be'. He returns to the
same theme when writing of Santa Maria in Monte: 'the majority both of the dead and of the sick are cacochymic, full of many
bad humours; they are poor people who eat food of bad quality
and for that reason many have died. It is our opinion that to protect these people from contracting these illnesses, since the
majority of them are poor, they should be provided with proper
food, since there are many of them who do not have bread and
die of want.'[42] Master mason Bastiano Brunelli, who had been
sent to Santa Maria in Monte to check whether the tombs were
adequately made, reached the same conclusion: 'if many poor
people had enough bread to feed themselves there would not be
so many sick.'[43]

Dr Ruschi's report dated 29 March 1612 ended on a reassuring
note: 'there is no need to be worried as there are not many sick.
Between the town *castello* and the plain there are about twenty
sick, which is not many.' But in the following August, Santa
Maria was engulfed by a new wave of disease, this time con-
sisting of malarial and dysenteric illnesses. On 25 September
1612 Dr Del Dua, the community doctor, wrote that 'since the
beginning of August and today there have been more than
twenty-five people sick in Santa Maria in Monte, but not all
have received treatment. The sicknesses were pure tertian fevers,
intermittent and continuous tertian fevers with much putrefaction and some dysenteric fluxes which are very hard to treat,
caused by the great heat and fatigue which inflamed the bile and
produced these various illnesses.'[44]

In the spring of 1613 it was the turn of Empoli and Montelupo.
On 14 April Giovan Battista Cocchi, a physician practising in
Empoli, reported that 'at present in Empoli I have in my care 15
patients, men and women, who are confined to bed, and are
suffering from simple and double bastard tertian fevers and for
the moment there is no sign of any malignant illness here. Outside the walls and for two or three miles round about there are
the same sicknesses but among them some cases of diarrhoea,
which are of bad quality but respond to treatment.' The other
doctor in Empoli, Piero Conti, wrote on the same day that 'I

have between 35 and 40 patients in my care and all live within a seven-mile radius of here, but half of them are from Empoli and especially from Montelupo where there is more hardship; and I have good hopes that all will recover since it is a sickness that only rarely becomes dangerous.'[45]

With the arrival of the summer the epidemic spread to other places. In a letter dated 12 August 1613 the Florentine Magistracy showed its awareness that 'there are many poor people who are sick and every day a considerable number of them are dying' in San Casciano, Barberino di Val d'Elsa, Poggibonsi, Certaldo, Castelfiorentino, Montelupo and Empoli.[46]

On 16 August the same Dr Cocchi who had reported from Empoli in April wrote that 'this morning I visited Montelupo and observed the sick in this community who amount to twenty men and women with perhaps about twelve children. The sicknesses are simple and double, that is bastard tertian fevers. Up to now they do not appear malignant and they respond well to treatment.'[47]

On 6 September Dr Cocchi sent another report. He recalled that in his previous report he had affirmed that 'the sicknesses were mild and responded to treatment because they were simple and double tertian fevers'. But in the meantime the situation seemed to have changed. 'From the middle of the past month of August until now there have been some fevers which have been malignant and at present there are six patients with malignant fever and they are in danger of their lives: and these patients are among the most prominent people in this *castello*. The first symptoms are acute head pains with continuous vomiting, and treatment is not effective.' Having said this, Dr Cocchi felt obliged to add that 'there are many other men, women and children who are not receiving treatment and I can therefore not give definite information about them, but it does not seem to me that many of the sick die'.[48] At the time, Montelupo must have had about five hundred inhabitants.[49]

In the summer of 1613 a malaria epidemic had also struck Castelfiorentino. A report by Giovanni Ronconi, a physician there, dated 19 August, gives an account of the episode. The doctor wrote: 'At the beginning of last July people in these areas and neighbouring communities where I practise began to fall sick of double tertian fevers, mostly intermittent, which on being treated passed without further harm to the patients. This continued until the end of the month, at which time greater numbers of people fell sick, they too suffering from two tertian fevers which were continuous because of overlapping; and a few die but most recover quickly. There are no *accidenti* symptoms except for continuous pains in the head and kidneys and great thirst, as one would expect from the fever and the summer season. Among these there have been and still are very few who are suffering from a tertian fever which strengthens every third day in accordance with its nature. In these cases one finds signs of malignity since they do not suffer from head- or other aches, as usually happens, they do not suffer great thirst, they do not appear to have a raging temperature, the urine of some is moderately good and their pulse fairly even. This *accidente* only occurs at the beginning of their sickness when their strength deserts them precipitously and their pulses and bodies remain very weak and some die in six days, others in ten or eleven.'[50]

As a supplement to Dr Ronconi's report the Podestà of Castelfiorentino sent the Florentine Magistracy a 'list of the sick', which shows that on 16 August 1613 there were:[51]

sick in Castelfiorentino	33	Nicolaio	8
San Matteo	3	Pieve S. Ippolito	2
Sant'Andrea a Montirandi	3	S. Piero a Pisangeli	1
Listra	4		

It seems therefore that morbidity was high. Mortality, on the other hand, was relatively low. The surviving death register for Castelfiorentino confirms Dr Ronconi's report to the letter. As we have seen, he reported that the epidemic had begun 'at the beginning of July' but that the fevers 'on being treated passed without further harm to the patients'. At the end of July 'greater numbers of people fell sick, they too suffering from tertian fevers . . . and some die of this but most recover quickly'. The following figures are derived from the surviving parish death register:[52]

Deaths

		adults	children	total
	September	2	–	2
1612	August	2	–	2
	September	2	–	2
	October	4	1	5
	November	3	–	3
	December	2	–	2
1613	January	1	–	1
	February	–	–	–
	March	2	–	2
	April	3	1	4
	May	1	–	1
	June	–	–	–
	July	–	1	1
	August	6	1	7
	September	5	2	7

In July, in spite of the widespread sickness, the number of deaths
(1) was actually lower than the monthly average during the
eleven preceding months (2). In the months of August and September the mortality curve rose steeply and the number of
deaths more than trebled (7) compared to the average of the
twelve preceding months (1.92). But these were still negligible
levels,[53] so that we must agree with the doctor that 'most [of the
patients] quickly recover'.

In 1615 it was the turn of Bibbona on the Tyrrhenian coast. We
do not know what rumours or information had reached the Florentine Magistracy, but the result was that the physician Dr
Perinto Collodi was sent on an inspection. Dr Collodi wrote his
report on 8 May 1615. According to this report, 'in this place
during the current year, namely from January until now, about
60 adults and children have died and at present there are only
seven or eight sick'. Only twenty-five of those who died,

however, were locals, 'who had been infected long ago and had been sick for a long time'. Most of the dead had been 'foreigners from Lombardy who had set out at the end of October and November to return home because of the sickness they had contracted in other places and since it seemed to them while passing through Bibbona that they had recovered, they stopped there with others of their countrymen to work while they were still convalescent, weak, suffering from an obstruction in the flow of their humours and liquids, showing the signs of cacochimia. These factors, combined with the continuous blowing of the scirocco for many months, caused them to fall ill.'

The doctor is referring here to the phenomenon of seasonal workers who moved from Northern Italy to the Tuscan Maremma year after year during the agricultural season. In the north there was high demographic pressure with relatively abundant labour. In the Tuscan Maremma, on the other hand, labour was relatively scarce because of malaria. This discrepancy gave rise to the migration of sizeable groups of agricultural workers, who moved temporarily to the Maremma in spring and summer to earn a crust of bread, frequently losing their lives there. The term 'Lombards' which Dr Collodi uses is inexact, however: the workers came from Liguria and above all from Emilia.[54]

As for the diseases which had caused the deaths referred to, the doctor reported that 'according to what the inhabitants told me they were putrid and malignant fevers, as they told me the sick suffered from delirium, thirst, restlessness, cloudy urine and stinking excrement, and finally exanthema or petechiae appeared on the skin. In addition many of those who died suffered inflammation of the pleura, commonly called *mal di punta* [stitch]. At present the sickness is absent and from what I hear in the Comune all those who took purgative and other medicines survived, having been treated by the Physicians of Volterra. These illnesses were not and are not contagious and in some houses people fell sick and died without infecting others who lived or visited there.'

The doctor concluded that 'at present things are in a good state' but recommended that orders be given 'to pave the streets, to clean the stables and to prohibit for some time the keeping of cattle, buffalos, pigs and geese inside the town'. In addition, 'since Bibbona is subject to disease because of its situation', Dr Collodi recommended 'that the Comune provide a doctor and a chemist since they are obliged to go for what they need to Volterra, which is so far that death arrives before the remedy'.

We have already seen that twenty-five locals, 'both adults and children', had died between the beginning of January and the beginning of May. Since the little town of Bibbona numbered perhaps fewer than one thousand souls, the level of mortality during the epidemic was equivalent to an annual rate of eighty per thousand. Following the Hippocratic tradition, Dr Collodi laid emphasis on geographical and meteorological factors among the causes of morbidity: 'The air is bad, not only because of the situation of the place which is low-lying and overshadowed by the nearby mountains, but also because it opens towards the damp southern winds.' And last but not least there was the usual problem of refuse: 'To this must be added a very obvious cause, the filthiness of the place, which is not paved and therefore produces vast quantities of mud and because of the unevenness of the terrain it is only with great difficulty that the inhabitants can remove the heaps of waste especially in the summer when it is very dry. What is worse and seems to be an important factor is that in the winter buffalos, cattle, pigs and geese are brought into the stables in the town and fill the stalls with manure which is not removed because of the scarcity of people and which causes infection.'[55]

In the second half of the second decade of the seventeenth century, exanthematous typhus, which was endemic in Italy, spread in an increasingly epidemic form. The Marche were particularly badly affected,[56] and it was probably from the Marche that typhus arrived in Florence. The Health Magistracy had been monitoring the situation with increasing concern for some time but did not sound the alarm until 17 December 1620. On that date the Magistracy sent the Grand-Duke a report in which it explained that 'for some time we have been observing week after week the number of deaths both in the homes and in the hospitals of the city; and we find that there is a significant number, over 130 per week, and for this reason we met today and discussed this business'.[57] The Florentine epidemic died down at the beginning of summer 1621 but flared up again in the spring of 1622 and lasted until the end of the following spring.[58] During this period the Magistrates were extremely active in taking various measures aimed at containing the effects of the epidemic in Florence,[59] but this did not prevent them from concerning themselves with the spread of the disease through the territories of the state.

By about the middle of January 1621 typhus had spread to Prato. The *castello*, including the outlying areas, numbered about 11,000 souls. According to the report which the Podestà sent to the Florentine Magistracy, in mid-February there were 'about 38 sick, mostly with petechiae, many of whom are in danger of their lives and 23 of whom are being treated by these doctors'. In addition there were 32 patients in the hospitals, that is '12 men and 20 women who are not very sick and whose illness is caused rather by deprivation than anything else as it is easy to see they are famished'. In the period between 1 and 15 February, 54 people died in the *castello*, 'both young and old'. Another 17 died between the 16th and the 23rd. In March 49 people died, seven of them in the hospital. In April 55 people died, 14 of them in the hospital, 'mostly of petechial sickness'. In May there were 47 deaths, ten of them in the hospital: 'most of those in the hospital died of old age and privation caused by poverty; but most of the others died of petechial disease which is very prevalent and very many are sick with this disease but many survive.'[60]

When the epidemic was still in its early stages, in the middle of February, the Podestà 'had both doctors set down in writing a description of the disease and its *accidenti*' in order to send reliable information to the Florentine Magistracy. There were two doctors practising in Prato: Dr Bernardino Gaci and Dr Giulio Bargellini. According to Dr Gaci – who judging from his handwriting must have been very old – 'for the past month there have been very many people sick with malignant tertian fevers and other fevers; with these fevers some burned inside and outside appeared quite cool, while others burned outside and were cold inside, and others felt cold in some parts of their bodies and hot in others; so that many died of these bad fevers'. In Dr Gaci's opinion this epidemic 'derived not only from the recent famine amongst the poor people and gluttony on the part of the citizens, but also from the heavenly bodies and from the fact that superior constellations influenced the inferior ones; so that these terrible fevers which resisted all treatment had many causes'. As for the 'contagiousness' of the disease, Dr Gaci wrote that 'there were no signs [of contagiousness]' and added in support of his thesis that 'those who work in the hospital and look after the sick have not suffered at all'. He concluded that 'nevertheless these sick-nesses this year have been more perverse, more wicked, more malignant'.[61]

The other doctor practising in Prato was Dr Giulio Bargellini. His report begins with the observation that 'since the 15th of January last many more people have fallen sick and died than is usual, most of whom were attacked by putrid and continuous fevers with certain indications of malignity and bad behaviour. The symptoms and *accidenti* which followed these fevers have been as follows: first a gentle and pleasant heat in the external parts which hardly differed from the normal, so that many were four days into the sickness before they consulted a doctor. Con-trasting with this heat were *accidenti* such as constant restless-ness, dryness and frequently blackness of the tongue, insatiable thirst, headaches, wakefulness, delirium, unequal heat between the viscera and the external parts of the body, the latter not being hot, the former being continuously burning hot. In most cases the pulse is weak, rapid, frequent and not without irreg-ularities while the urine is cloudy, dark and smelly. Furthermore on many patients petechiae of varied colour and quantity appeared before the seventh and up to the eleventh and seven-teenth [days]. However, from what we have seen up to now (God be praised) the fevers do not appear to be contagious, since it has rarely happened that more than one person is sick of these types of illness in a house at any one time; and in particular in the hospital, where if this were the case there would have been certain proof; and up to now this has not happened.'

As for 'the causes of these kinds of illness, although it is not
easy to discover the truth', the doctor mentioned 'the changeable
weather during the past and present season, the errors com-
mitted in the six non-natural things,* the bad disposition of those
bodies which have been affected, the hardship and famine which
the poor and low-class people seem to suffer from and perhaps
some malign celestial influence'. As for the mortality caused by
the disease, Dr Bargellini reported that 'of those on whom petechiae appeared before the seventh [day] few survived and most
died around the ninth or eleventh day and before the fourteenth,
and those who survived the fourteenth almost all recovered'. Regarding the treatments used, Dr Bargellini wrote that 'great care
has been taken and observations made to change and vary all
types of remedies both in quantity and kind and method of use;
but up to now there has been no certain, trustworthy conclusion
about any of the methods except to say that those who ate well at
the beginning of the illness and during it were much more likely
to recover than those who lived and ate more frugally'.[62]

The territories in the Val d'Arno bordering on the Marche gave
particular cause for concern. On 20 April 1622 the Magistrates
wrote to the Grand Duke: 'Certain news has been received in the
city that in many places in the Marche and particularly the Holy
House of Loreto, Recanati, Macerata, Fermo and other places in
that area are prey to dangerous and contagious illnesses.' In
view of this information the Magistrates informed the Grand
Duke that 'we have attended to this by writing to the Capitano of
Borgo San Sepolcro, the official of this state who is nearest that
area, to take steps to discover the truth'. In the same letter they
wrote that 'we have also heard that in the Val d'Arno above San
Giovanni and Montevarchi and around there many people are
sick and many dying'.[63] Three days later the Magistrates informed the Grand Duke that they had written to 'the Capitano of
Borgo [San Sepolcro] and then to the Vicario of San Giovanni
[to] the Podestà of Figline and [the one at] Montevarchi by fast

---

* The six non-natural things are: air, food, sleep, motion, excretion and affections of the
mind.

messenger' asking for urgent news about the local health situation. In those decades the administration worked well and the Magistrates were able to write to the Grand Duke that 'the answers have returned with the reports which we enclose'.[64] In fact the archive contains the reports of the Capitano of Borgo San Sepolcro (19 April), the Vicario of San Giovanni (21 and 24 April), the Podestà of Montevarchi (22 April) and of Dr Antonio Durazzini who practised in Figline and wrote on behalf of the Podestà of Figline and on his instructions (21 April).

In his letter dated 21 April to the Florentine Magistracy the Vicario of San Giovanni wrote that having received 'your welcome letter by fast messenger I immediately called in Messer Latanzio Magiotti who is the physician here ... and you will find his report enclosed'. Unfortunately there is no trace of Dr Magiotti's report, which is a pity because Magiotti was an interesting man. He was born of a patrician family in Montevarchi in 1590 and graduated in medicine and philosophy in Pisa in 1612. In 1622 he was community doctor in San Giovanni. In 1630 he was community doctor in Prato. He then went to Florence where he obtained a brilliant position: he numbered Galileo among his patients and was made physician to the Grand-Ducal court.[65] Dr Magiotti seems to have been an advocate of 'therapeutic nihilism': in other words he was decidedly sceptical of the therapeutic capabilities of medicine and the therapeutic properties of the medicines of his time. According to Count Lorenzo Magalotti, 'our dear friend Magiotti said quite openly [that doctors and medicines were useless] and when Grand Duke Ferdinand asked how in all honesty he could accept money from patients knowing he could not cure them he replied: "Most Serene Highness, I take the money not for my services as a doctor but as a guard, to prevent some young man who believes everything he reads in books from coming along and stuffing something down the patients which kills them." '[66]

The Capitano of Borgo San Sepolcro had no medical training but his report is clear and precise and leaves no doubt about the presence of exanthematous typhus in the town. From his own declarations ('The doctor believes ...') we know that the Capitano consulted the local doctor before writing his report.

According to what the Capitano wrote, 'the nature of the present sicknesses is as follows: continuous malignant fevers accompanied by extraordinary *accidenti* and contagious through close contact. They begin with a slight heat which increases somewhat in the evening until the fourth hour and then disappears. The pulse immediately becomes very weak and although they do not become delirious until the seventh or ninth [day] nevertheless they are not completely rational and during this period they ramble without becoming angry, recalling their affairs and if questioned they return to normal for a while. After two or three days the urine of most patients has a deposit like flour which is almost the colour of ash. Until the fourth [day] they have difficulty in eating, with some vomiting; on the sixth [day] the tongue becomes black and, in some, spotted in various places with drips of blood from the nose; on the sixth [day] petechiae of all kinds appear and disappear on the torso. Many experience an emptying of the bowels and pass a great quantity of urine on the eleventh or thirteenth [day] and with these the delirium finishes and with their pulse continuing weak they die on the sixteenth, or twelfth or fourteenth [day] affirming that they do not feel anything weighing on them. All those who die are either dissolute or incontinent, or full of troublesome thoughts. At present there are four or five of these patients. There are several others with various strange sicknesses such as fluxes of urine, spasms, vomiting, chest pains.' As usual there were also some people suffering from intermittent malaria-type fevers: 'the doctor says he has patients with simple and double tertian fevers, which are not very long-lasting and intermittent, and all of these recover. Children, women and old people mostly recover and all those who recover empty their bowels.'

According to the Capitano, 'about 5,000 people live in this town'. As for the number of deaths, there were 366 between 1 May 1621 and 19 April 1622.[67] The Capitano does not state whether the figure he provides includes children or not. If they are included, the general mortality rate on an annual basis was about 76 per thousand. If childhood deaths were not counted, however, the general mortality rate was obviously much higher.

As has been said, Dr Antonio Durazzini, the local community doctor, reported on the health situation in Figline. According to Durazzini, 'the sicknesses are intermittent and continuous tertian fevers, many tertian fevers which become continuous at the third bout and malignant with cloudy urine and weak pulse, which I believe to be caused by a superabundance of all the humours but especially the bilious ones, caused not only by the bad weather which has been very unsettled and unseasonable for the past two years but also by the disorderly, wicked way of life in all the six non-natural things. I do not think these illnesses are contagious since not only those who visit the sick but even those who live in the same house do not fall ill. There is no apparent fever. There is no corruption of the limbs or *accidenti* (though some have petechiae) associated with pestilential fevers as I have seen on other occasions.

'The *accidenti* of these illnesses are headache, lassitude and pains all over in all the torso, unquenchable thirst, delirium, somnolence, petechiae (but only in a few cases), sweating, bilious bowel movements, and most of those who died did so on the fourteenth [day] or after, from loss of strength caused by the persistent feverish heat. At the moment I have ten patients in my care (five women and the same number in the hospital) suffering from continuous fevers due to angina. How many there are in the place as a whole I do not know.

'The sacristan of the parish church, who has been keeping count from 3 February [1622] until today [21 April] tells me that there have been 29 deaths in the town and in the hospital, of whom twelve were old people between seventy and ninety years old and of those who were sick I treated six.'

As for treatments, Dr Durazzini mentioned 'in the first place the emission of blood [that is, blood-letting] and soothing medicament before the seventh day'. He then listed 'other medicines for internal and external use'. Among the medicines for internal use he listed: citron juice syrup and conserve, hyacinth electuary, jewel alkermes, cold daisy electuary, salsify fever water, jewelled juleb, bezoar stone and contrienna. 'But above all jewelled juleb, salsify water and fever water.' Among externally applied medicines he mentions poultices to the heart, anti-venomous oil, baths of the genitals and feet, vesicants and cupping glasses. And he ended with a note which would have delighted Dr Latanzio Magiotti: 'More of those who are able to seek medical advice and treatment die than of the poor.'[68]

The reply from Montevarchi came directly from the Podestà, who did, however, repeat the opinion of the local doctor: 'The doctor says that for several months past there have been many people here sick with acute fever, some [fevers] with petechiae but most without, some with delirium, and other *accidenti* which tend to accompany malignant fevers. Some died under treatment but most recovered. At present there are three sick with malignant fevers, all inside the town; and a few others suffering from sporadic sickness.'

When the Podestà wrote his report the area was in the grip of a severe famine. After the abundant harvest of 1612 Tuscans had enjoyed cheap bread for about four years. In Siena the price of bread fell below 70 *soldi* a *staio** in September 1612 to a low of 58 *soldi* in April–May 1616. After this the situation changed. The 1616 harvest was meagre, those of 1617, 1618 and 1619 were pitiful. In 1620 the harvest was quite good and contemporaries described it as 'reasonable', but the harvest of the following year, 1621, was literally disastrous. As a result, from March 1617 the price of a *staio* of grain on the Siena market stayed above 70 *soldi* and in May–June 1620 rose to 119 soldi, reaching 120 *soldi* in June 1622. One of the last observations made in the Podestà of Montevarchi's report should be read in the light of this situation: 'As for the countryside there has been less sickness and fewer have died, some of them of hunger: not that food is lacking, but it's too dear for them to buy.'[69] Clearly the Podestà was not well versed in economics.

As we have already seen, Dr Latanzio Magiotti's report on Borgo San Giovanni cannot be found at present. However, the doctor's conclusions are briefly summarised in a report written by the Podestà, dated 24 April 1622: 'almost all the patients have petechiae and go crazy and some survive seven days, some fourteen or a little more.'[70]

---

* 1 staio = about 17 kilograms.

To conclude, of the four centres which concerned the Florentine Magistracy (Borgo San Sepolcro, Borgo San Giovanni, Figline and Montevarchi), in two (Borgo San Sepolcro and Borgo San Giovanni) typhus had reached epidemic proportions while in the other two (Figline and Montevarchi) there seem to have been only a few isolated cases. However, all things considered, the situation was not a cheerful one and it is astonishing to read in the report sent by the Magistrates to the Grand Duke that 'We have shown these reports to Dr Zerbinelli, who serves our office, and it seems that there is nothing to worry about and that the sicknesses have been and are of the same type which have been going around and still are going around in other parts of the state and the city of Florence.'

Meanwhile the Florentine Magistracy had received news of widespread sickness in Pieve S. Stefano 'and that people are dying of contagious illnesses and therefore they desire to know what kind of illnesses there are, the *accidenti* which have occurred and the number of deaths in recent times'. They therefore requested Dr Stefano Ronbelli, the local doctor, to write a report. Dr Ronbelli wrote his report in May 1622:

'I can therefore tell you that since the beginning of May many people have been ill, not all with the same illness, however some have suffered from simple and double tertian fevers, some from catarrh, some from malignant fevers and petechiae and the numbers have varied from 20 to 25 and finally 30.

'If I remember rightly, eight people have died since the beginning of May, that is, a woman of 65 who died of various indispositions and catarrh, a man of 40 suffering from catarrh in the throat who died quite suddenly, a 60-year-old man of malignant fever and petechiae, a man of almost the same age of the same illness, another woman of about 50 of malignant fever with petechiae, a woman of childbirth, another woman of the same thing, a boy of 14 who had been ill for six years and died of consumption.'

According to Dr Ronbelli, 'those who have survived malignant fevers and petechiae – and there have been many, thanks to the treatments used – had bowel movement on the critical day and several days after and were then free of the disease. Some sweated and some passed urine. In short in those with defects, despite all the treatments, their languid vitality could not pass on [the properties of the medicaments] through critical movement and the patients died. But they were a small number compared to the total number of sick. Now the number of patients seems to have dropped off. The *accidenti* which occurred during the malignant fevers were, in some, great thirst with blackened tongue, thick and reddish urine, headaches, weakness in the whole body and pain in legs and bones. Some suffered delirium. The *accidenti* during convalescence were: some went deaf, some could hardly see, others were almost crazy but in a short space of time everything was sorted out and [the patients returned] to full health.'[71]

There could also be false alarms. One occurred in 1623. We do not know how the Florentine Magistracy received news of exceptionally high morbidity and mortality levels in Santa Sofia. The Magistrates immediately instructed Giovanni Malvisi, a physician practising in Bagnio, to go to Santa Sofia and inform the Magistracy about the nature and seriouness of the events. When he got there the doctor naturally found some sick people, but within normal limits: 'I found seven in all, among them Fabritio the son of the doctor, Messer Vincentio Gentili, who is convalescing under his father's care from an attack of melancholy.' Out of a population of 'about 600 souls' the number of sick appeared normal: not much over 1 per cent. 'Santa Sofia,' wrote the doctor, 'is a healthy place: good air, good food and as far as I can discover no one has suffered from any contagious illness for many years.'[72]

Dr Malvisi concludes on a humorous note: 'I was well received and when I left the chief townspeople accompanied me beyond the bridge. I saw people who were lively with good colour and without fear. In fact they were amazed that such a rumour had spread and pleased that their masters [that is, the Grand Dukes] were so solicitous towards them.'[73]

Dr Francesco Figlinesi found a very different situation in Castelfiorentino when he was sent there on inspection by the Florentine Magistracy in 1627. On 1 October he wrote the following report: 'In accordance with Your Lordships' [of the Magistracy] instructions I spoke at length – in the presence of Signor Attavanti the parish priest and Signor Guiducci the Provveditore who took part in every treatment – to the doctor of Castelfiorentino about the nature, conditions, *accidenti* and causes of the sickness which began to afflict these people in the late summer and early autumn and continues to do so. Thirty people have died between August 22nd and September 30th and of 500 adults living in this place, both rich and poor, 150 or so have fallen sick: according to the doctor who has treated them and observed them carefully they have suffered from two types of illness. Some have had a sickness which was bad right from the beginning, causing immediate loss of strength and fever which was clearly continuous, followed by marking of the skin with tiny marks like flea bites, restlessness, dryness of the tongue and urine not much different from the nature of the sickness. The result was that as the sickness worsened many of these, being greatly weakened, died on the seventh, eleventh or fourteenth day of sickness according to their powers of natural resistance. The excrements show more or less signs of sickness which is accompanied by more or less severe *accidenti*; the time of death did not exceed two weeks after the onset of the acute illness.

'In two of the patients at present under observation the sickness followed a different course from in other cases since, not having had the outbreak of tertian fever which occurred three times, they suddenly fell asleep with evident offence to the animal faculty, remaining without motion or feeling in any part of the body, with spots on the skin as above, difficulty in breathing, without eating, so that we believe they will shortly die since their strength cannot resist such damage; and the worst of it is that one of them has not taken communion and the other is a woman who is without the sacrament of confession although every possible help is being given.

'The other kind of sickness has been double tertian fevers which have not shown themselves to be, nor do they appear to be, of bad nature but are rather resistant to treatment, depending most of them on the abundant soaking of the viscera which recognisably suffer from hardness and notable tensions.

'It has been observed that in addition to those fevers many people are suffering from the disease of the weights (gastrointestinal infections) and although people of all ranks suffer, nevertheless more poor people have it because of the bad food they eat; and since this sickness seems to be of a contagious nature and is easily caught it happens that in some houses three or four people are suffering from this illness and most do not treat it because they cannot afford to, but leave everything to nature.'

From the epidemiological point of view, Dr Figlinesi noted 'that almost all those who fell sick lived on this side of the bridge and in this part of town in one street more than any of the others, and among the sick there are more well-off than poor people'.

Dr Figlinesi attributed the origin of the epidemic above all to the prevailing filth: 'After careful examination we believe the causes of the sicknesses to be the impurity and foulness of the air followed by the filth of manure and heaps of fertilisers which can be found in the houses of the peasants lodging in the *castello* as well as the fact that they have stabled large and small animals together in the same place, and themselves live in old houses which give off foul odours and stenches which you can smell even just walking through the place without entering the houses. In addition to this disorder [is] the fact that butchers do their work in the centre of the *castello*.' Dr Figlinesi followed the Hippocratic tradition in not neglecting the geophysical element: 'Consider the location and position of the place which for the most part looks south from west and consequently is very subject to southern and sea winds and since most of the houses are on the hillside and do not have any outlet to the back, it happens that the houses are penetrated by the winds in greater measure and by the harmful vapours created by the action of heat on the filth which, as we have already said, is kept around the houses.'[74]

In his report Dr Figlinesi writes that the population of Castelfiorentino numbered about 500 adults, which means a total population of 800 or 900. On 22 September the number of adult sick was put at 72.[75] But then subsidies arrived from Florence for the sick poor and, as Commissario Guiducci noted, 'When this money was distributed and the poor visited in their homes it was found that there were many sick people who were not on the doctor's list since, being poor and unable to pay for medicines, they are left to the care of nature and do not call the doctor.'[76] At the end of September the actual number of sick was reckoned at about 150 adults; more than a quarter of the population. According to Dr Figlinesi, 30 people died between 22 August and 30 September. Castelfiorentino's parish register of the dead reveals that 21 adults and 9 'children' died.[77] Therefore between 22 August and 30 September the total mortality (that is, inclusive of 'children') reached a level which on an annual basis would have been over 300 per thousand.

On 19 October Dr Figlinesi had returned to Florence where he lived and practised and wrote 'from home' to the Magistracy informing them that 'on the secretary's order I left Castelfiorentino, where I left the people in universally good health, there being only a few sick with seasonal illnesses such as quartan fevers and catarrhs. The others who were ill previously are sure to recover soon and are making good progress. The whole inspection took me twenty-one days.'[78]

Chapter 4

Doctors, Diseases and the People

As we saw in Chapter 1, the Health Magistracy was primarily concerned with plague and the Magistrates' activities were directed mainly towards the prevention of the outbreak of a plague epidemic. However, while reading the texts of the medical reports reproduced in Chapter 3, the reader will have noticed that one of the first questions asked by the Magistracy's envoys on arrival in the places they inspected was whether any 'petechiae or other bad sign' had appeared on the bodies of patients there. This might lead the reader to believe that the Magistracy and its envoys were concerned not with plague but with petechial typhus. Such a conclusion would be erroneous, however, and would reflect modern medical knowledge and ways of thinking which are totally alien to the period we are dealing with.

Seventeenth-century doctors had no knowledge of microbes, viruses and vectors; they were misled in their clinical judgements by the humoral and miasmatic paradigms; they lacked the support provided by laboratory analysis; and their notions of disease classification were therefore inevitably confused. The concept of a disease as a specific entity was vague and imprecise and limited to a very few pathological forms; similarly, the doctrine of etiological specificity had not yet become part of medical knowledge. Diseases were frequently categorised on the basis of their lethality. So Fracastoro wrote, for example, that 'Sunt et aliae febres quam mediae quommodo sunt inter vere pestilentes et non pestilentes quoniam ab iis multi quidem pereunt multi etiam evadunt': he was referring to exanthematous typhus. In addition there was a widespread belief that a non-pestilential fever could be transformed into a pestilential fever if the environmental conditions on which the nature and seriousness of the disease depended deteriorated. This explains why, in the middle of the severe epidemic of exanthematous typhus which was raging in Florence in the spring of 1621, the Health Magistrates were able to declare with evident satisfaction in a letter to the Grand-Duke that the measures taken had 'until now preserved this city from contagion'.[1] Evidently the Magistrates did not consider the typhus epidemic to be a 'contagion': 'contagion' meant an epidemic of plague and there was no plague in Florence in 1621.

Exanthematous typhus, or as it was called then 'malignant fever with *accidenti*, of petechiae', was regarded as a pathological state with rather high mortality. During the period covered by the medical reports included in the previous chapter the plague was absent from Italy. Exanthematous thyphus, however, was very prevalent. It is therefore not surprising that the doctors sent by the Magistracy were anxious to find out whether petechiae had appeared in the places they visited. If there were petechiae it meant that a dangerous level of 'malignity' had been reached, which in turn meant that the fevers might lead to 'contagion' i.e. to the plague. The spectre of plague was always at the back of everyone's mind.

The doctors of the period were obviously interested in assessing the 'contagiousness' and lethality of the various nosological categories which had been more or less vaguely identified. The science of statistics had not yet been born; and even if some doctors made use of mortality figures, generally in a rough and ready way, lethality was not calculated in terms of precise numerical probability. It was sufficient to refer to 'malignant' and 'pestilential' forms to indicate those illnesses whose outcome was frequently fatal. Obviously the plague came first in the league of malignity.

When the doctor from Pietrasanta was sent to Massa in September 1623 to assess the local public health situation, he wrote to the Magistrates reassuring them that it was not plague, because 'plague', wrote the doctor, 'tends to kill the majority while these are more alive than dead'.[2] As for 'contagiousness', the plague was also regarded as the contagious disease *par excellence*, so much so that as we have seen in the passage already cited from the letter written by the Florentine Magistrates to the Grand Duke, the term 'contagion' was used as a synonym for plague (see p. 67).

In 1546 G. Fracastoro had included petechial fevers in his treatise *De contagiosis morbis*, but seventeenth-century doctors were continually perplexed by the contagiousness of these fevers. They were ignorant of the cause of the illness and its method of diffusion. Their only point of reference was the haemorrhagic suffusions known as petechiae. But petechiae are common to various diseases including (though infrequently) malaria.[3] In 1608 during the malaria epidemic which raged through the Florentine state, according to Dr Bernardini in Santa Maria in Monte, in various cases of 'simple and double tertian fever . . . on the fourth or seventh [day] petechiae appear in some people'. In the same year during the same epidemic in Fucecchio, Dr Guidoni reported that petechiae appeared on four patients but that 'since relatives and helpers frequented the same rooms and indeed slept in the same bed without falling ill', he concluded that there was no 'contagion' (p. 30). The petechiae seen by Dr Bernardini in Santa Maria in Monte and by Dr Guidoni on four patients in Fucecchio were possibly caused by malarial infection, which would explain why the four people in Fucecchio did not transmit 'petechial fevers' to those who had slept with them 'in the same bed' (given that prevailing sanitary conditions meant that there was no lack of lice).

We saw earlier that in the early phases of the typhus epidemic which occurred in Prato in 1621 Dr Gaci, one of the two local doctors, observed that 'no signs [of contagiousness] have been seen' (see p. 55). This surprising observation was based fundamentally on the fact that no one among the patients or workers in the hospital had caught the disease: 'those who work in the hospital and look after the sick have not suffered at all'. On the same date, the other doctor in Prato, Dr Bargellini, wrote that 'from what we have seen up to now (God be praised) the fevers do not appear to be contagious since it has rarely happened that more than one person is sick of these types of illness in a house at any one time and in particular in the hospital, where if this were the case there would have been certain proof and up to now this has not happened'.

Clearly in mid-February 1621 both Dr Gaci and Dr Bargellini believed that the disease was not infectious since there had not been a series of cases in the hospital. If typhus had in fact penetrated the hospital in Prato it would have been very strange for it not to have spread rapidly among the patients. The hospitals of the time were full of lice as well as fleas, bedbugs and other unpleasant insects; and there is no reason to believe that the hospital in Prato was an exception. The explanation for the relative healthiness of Prato hospital in mid-February 1621 must be sought elsewhere. At that time, hospitals took in sick people only incidentally. In normal times the hospital took in above all the very poor who had nothing to eat and nowhere to sleep. In one of the Podestà of Prato's reports we read that the 32 patients in the hospital in mid-February 'are not very ill and their illness is caused rather by deprivation than anything else, as it is easy to see they are famished'. It is reasonable to assume, therefore, that in the middle of February typhus had not yet penetrated the hospital and that the patients were there solely because of poverty. This would explain the absence of a chain of infection which gave the two doctors the pious illusion that the disease was not infectious (or, to use their vocabulary, 'contagious').

Malarial fevers were endemic to Tuscany and no one was particularly worried by them. In 1459 when Alessandra Macinghi Strozzi heard that her son Matteo, who was in exile with his brothers in Naples, had fallen ill, 'I was grief-stricken,' she wrote, 'and feared for his life.' But then 'I called Francesco and sent for Matteo di Giorgio and heard from both of them that his sickness was tertian fever so I took comfort because you do not die of tertian fever, unless other illnesses intervene'.[4] In this particular case her optimism was misplaced because Matteo Strozzi

died within the month, but as we have seen (p. 51) in the malaria
epidemic which struck Castelfiorentino in 1613, a high morbidity
rate was accompanied by decidedly low mortality.

In Liguria malarial fevers were regarded with much greater
suspicion than in Tuscany. Dr Monti, who was sent by the Florentine Magistracy to assess the nature of the epidemic which
was raging in the Genoese Republic in August 1632, was
astonished to find that the Genoese health authorities quaran-
tined in the pest-house on 'suspicion of infection' (*purga di sos-
petto*) people returning from the Maremma who, in the Tuscan
doctor's opinion, were suffering only from 'ordinary fevers'.[5]

The term 'disease of the weights' (*male di pondi*) was used to refer to gastro-intestinal infections in general, and so to a huge
range of infectious diseases excluding, however, cholera, which
appeared in Europe for the first time in the nineteenth century.
In 1627, as we have seen (p. 64), Dr Figlinesi wrote in his report
on Castelfiorentino that 'this illness [*male di pondi*] has a contagious nature and is easily caught; and so it happened that in
some houses three or four suffer from the said illness'. But it is
impossible to know what kind of infection Dr Figlinesi was referring to: he did not even know himself.

Influenza is a highly contagious disease. During the period
under discussion, and in Tuscan documents of the Health
Magistracy, the term 'influenza' did not indicate the illness as
we know it but rather a situation of increased morbidity whatever the disease (or diseases) which made up that morbidity.
What we call influenza today did not have a name because it was
not perceived as a specific, distinct entity. People spoke in
generic terms of catarrhs, illnesses of the chest and lungs, inflammations of the throat, pleurisy, referring to various manifes-
tations or pathological complications of the disease. The prevailing theory (see pp. 33 and 44) was that the catarrhs which
caused these illnesses derived from the 'phlegmatic humours'
which formed in people's brains as a result of the winter cold.
The idea of a climatological origin excluded de facto the idea of
contagion and it is interesting to recall what Dr Ruschi wrote on
the subject when he visited Santa Maria in Monte in 1612 in the
middle of what was probably a flu epidemic. Dr Ruschi com-

mented that 'the general opinion is that they are not contagious diseases but common sicknesses which affect now one place, now another, and God forbid they should be contagious as we should all be sick by now' (see p. 47).

The virus which in one patient produces a fever that lasts only three days can cause the death of another. In 1961 Eickhoff wrote that influenza is a disease characterised by high morbidity and low mortality. The lethality rate of influenza today rarely exceeds 0.01 per cent on average.[6]

The lethality of influenza is partly influenced by the nature of the virus and to a much greater degree by the patient's age, physiological condition and immunological history. There is practically no satisfactory documentary evidence on the physiological condition of rural Tuscans in the seventeenth century. Given this gap in our knowledge, the comments on the subject in the medical reports constitute precious evidence despite their incidental character, vagueness and lack of precise quantitative data. We have seen that on his visit to Campiglia in 1611 Dr Cesare Ruschi commented that 'we must consider that the majority of those who died were poor peasants who were exhausted by hard work and ill nourished, as the poor tend to be' (p. 45). The same Dr Ruschi, visiting Santa Maria in Monte in 1612, wrote that 'the majority both of the dead and of the sick are cacochymic, full of many bad humours: they are poor people who eat food of bad quality and for that reason many have died. It is our opinion that to protect these people from contracting these illnesses, since the majority of them are poor, they should be provided with proper food since there are many of them who do not have bread and die of want' (p. 48). It was reported from Montevarchi in 1622 that 'some [of the sick] died of hunger' (p. 60). In his report on Castelfiorentino in 1627 Dr Figlinesi wrote: 'many people are suffering from disease of the weights . . . more poor people have it because of the bad food they eat' (p. 64). The Florentine Magistracy was informed in a report from Tizzana in 1621 that 'sickness in these parts proceeds more from the great poverty of the people than from anything else because they lead a wretched life'.[7]

Feelings of humanitarian compassion such as we find in the

above comments might be accompanied by a sense of intelligent practicality, as in the recommendation made by Dr Giovanni Malvisi in 1623 that 'if there were sick people who were too poor to pay for medicine and food, they should be provided with what is necessary at public expense so that they do not infect the others'.[8]

The present-day lethality rate of 0.01 per cent for influenza is the result of the appropriate treatment that is available nowadays. Seventeenth-century patients did not have the benefit of modern treatments, however. The essential therapies to which physicians had recourse were blood-letting, purges and emetics (see pp. 32, 42, 43, 49, 88 n.29). Fortunately children were spared these lethal treatments (p. 43) but adults could not escape them. The results were deplorable. According to the experiments conducted by Dr Dietl in Vienna and Dr Bennett in Edinburgh in the nineteenth century the use of phlebotomies, purges and emetics in the treatment of broncho-pulmonary infections increased mortality by about two-thirds.

If we take together the poor physiological condition of the mass of the population and the counter-productive treatments used by doctors, we have to conclude that the lethality of influenza at the times and in the places we are dealing with must have been considerable. Events in Vico Pisano in 1610 may provide some indication. At the peak of an epidemic possibly of flu which struck Vico Pisano in that year, thirteen adults died during the month of April (pp. 29, 42), that is 5.6 times the monthly average (2.3 adult deaths) over the previous ten months.[9] Even if we allow that not all the deaths that occurred in that month of April were attributable to influenza, it is undeniable that it must have had a considerable effect on the general mortality.

The mass of the rural population was not inclined to seek medical treatment. First and foremost, given the widespread poverty, patients and their families were often unable to pay the doctor's fees. Furthermore, the physicians inspired feelings of reverent fear and peasants preferred to consult the local charlatan or wise woman. In the countryside around Fucecchio in 1608 there were 'many sick people who normally do not seek treatment for their illnesses' (p. 30) and 'most of them have not called the doctor, either because they are too poor or because they have little faith in medicine' (p. 32). At Santa Maria in Monte, struck by an epidemic of malarial fevers in 1608, 'few undergo treatment because of poverty or the scant faith they have in medicine' (p. 33). At San Miniato in the same year 'the peasants treat themselves and hardly ever consult the doctor either because they are too poor to pay for the treatment or because they have little faith in medicine, as is usual among country people' (pp. 34–5). At Marciana, Ponte Sacco and Bientina, which were struck by an influenza epidemic in 1610, the doctors reiterated monotonously that 'very few of the sick sought any treatment' (p. 37, 39, 40). At Campiglia in 1611, according to Dr Ruschi, 'most of the poor only send for the doctor when they need the priest' (p. 45). At Montelupo in 1613, according to Dr Cocchi, 'there are many other men, women and children who are not receiving treatment' (p. 49). At Castelfranco in 1627, according to Dr Figlinesi, '[the patients] being poor and unable to pay for medicines they are left to the care of nature and do not call the doctor' (p. 65).

It is difficult to say to what extent the peasants were really sceptical about the therapeutic powers of official medicine, as doctors continually asserted. I believe that the psychological resistance to seeking medical help owed more to economic factors than to a critical assessment of doctors' treatments. Such an assessment would have implied a degree of knowledge and analytical capacity which the majority of peasants certainly did not possess.[10] However, by avoiding doctors, poor people unwittingly protected themselves from practices which often more than doubled the probability of a fatal outcome. It comes as no surprise to read in Dr Durazzini's report on Figline in 1622 his candid statement on the subject, that 'more of those who are able to seek medical advice and treatment die than of the poor' (p. 60).

Chapter 5

Conclusion

Some time ago Dr M.D. Grmek observed that 'for too long historians and demographers have been bewitched by the spectacular devastation caused by plague and have therefore neglected the impact of other diseases. Among the exceptions we might mention the disasters caused by smallpox among the Amerindians during the sixteenth century, by cholera in the last century and by influenza in this.' Dr Grmek further observed that 'until very recent times the history of diseases has been studied almost exclusively in an analytical way, that is examining separately the history of separate diseases or groups of similar diseases'. Taking these considerations as his point of departure, Dr Grmek proposed a new, synthetic approach to the study of the history of disease and epidemiology; that is, one which considers the totality of pathological states present in a given population during a given historical period.[1] This is what I have tried to do in this short study for a large part of the area covered by the Florentine state, taking advantage of the existence of the medical reports to the Health Magistracy in Florence.

The Tuscan doctors who wrote the reports quoted above were hampered by many factors: lack of a systematic classification of diseases; absence of correct notions about the aetiological specificity of the various diseases; constant confusion between disease and symptoms and between infection and contagion; the misleading paradigms of humours and miasmas. Nevertheless they provided descriptions which, although unclear at some points, when taken together enable us to identify approximately the general pattern of morbidity which prevailed in the Florentine state in the early decades of the seventeenth century.

Between 1608 and 1628 plague was absent from the Florentine state (it returned in 1630). But, as we would expect in a pre-industrial society, the general pattern reveals a massive predominance of other infectious diseases, particularly influenza, malaria, petechial typhus and gastro-intestinal infections. These diseases were present in endemic form, breaking out into epidemics from time to time. The high morbidity which afflicted Fucecchio, Santa Maria in Monte, Castelfranco di sotto and San Miniato al Tedesco in 1608 was seemingly caused by an epidemic of malaria (see pp. 30–34). The epidemic which struck Florence in 1620–1, spread to Prato in 1621 (p. 54) and came from the Marche to rage through Borgo San Giovanni and Borgo San Sepolcro in 1621–2 (pp. 56–7) was an epidemic of exanthematous typhus. The sicknesses which occurred in Marciana, Cascina, Pontedera, Peccioli, Ponte a Sacco, San Pietro in Colle and Bientina in 1610 (pp. 36–40) were probably caused by an influenza epidemic which affected the whole of Europe in that year.[2] The high levels of morbidity and mortality in Santa Maria in Monte in 1612 (45ff) may also have been caused by an epidemic of influenza.

The epidemics of malaria, petechial typhus and influenza to which we have referred were accompanied by epidemic outbreaks of other diseases such as smallpox, otitis and mumps. At San Pietro in Collina in 1610, right in the middle of the flu epidemic, there was an outbreak of otitis media which in some cases led to complications of purulent infections ('many of them had great quantities of horrible discharge from their ears') (p. 40). At Campiglia in 1611, during an outbreak of respiratory tract infections, probably caused by an influenza epidemic, there was an outbreak of smallpox which, as we have seen (pp. 43–4), in the space of one month killed twenty children out of a community which cannot have numbered more than one thousand souls. Again in 1611 at Santa Maria in Monte, during an influenza epidemic, there was an epidemic of mumps which in some cases appears to have been fatal (p. 47). On the other hand various cases described in different reports as 'angina' may well have in fact been diphtheria. The description of cases in Borgo San Sepolcro in 1622 in which the urine presented 'a kind of flour at the bottom which is almost the colour of ash' leads us to suspect that these may have been cases of typhus, anthrax or hepatitis. With regard to hepatitis, one might suppose on a purely intuitive basis that it was not uncommon, given the indescribable filthiness which then prevailed. If this supposition is correct, one can only be astonished by the total absence from the medical reports of symptoms as easy to observe and describe as the abnormal coloration of tissue pigment.

Diseases do not develop in a vacuum. It would be a grave mistake to limit oneself to an aetiological concept of diseases which considers only the action of microbes or viruses. Microbes and viruses are the leading actors in the pathological drama. But epidemiological studies have made us increasingly aware of the role of environmental and socio-economic factors in the aetiology, incidence and prevalence of diseases. The fact that certain ages and certain cultures have been afflicted by the predominance of certain pathologies while other ages and other cultures suffer from others is both well established and significant. In pre-industrial societies, for example, there is an overwhelming prevalence of infectious pathologies, whereas degenerative pathologies prevail in industrial societies (but influenza seems to be the exception, striking both kinds of society without distinction). The pattern of morbidity in a given society is determined above all by socio-economic and hygienic conditions. Conversely the pattern of morbidity in a given society influences the economy of that society both directly and indirectly.

The disease which provoked the most shattering demographic shocks was the plague, with its very high mortality rate. Leaving aside the human aspects of a plague epidemic, the mortality *per se* was neither a good nor an evil. It all depended on the condition and structure of the economy. If the economy was trapped in a Malthusian-type situation with an excess of population in relation to the availability of capital, the elimination in the space of a few months of one-third or one-quarter of the population might have had positive effects. Obviously a precise analysis would have to take account of differential mortality between the various age groups and social groups. But it is obvious that after a plague epidemic the relationship between capital and labour generally shifted towards a greater availability of capital per unit of labour. On the other hand, if the demographic shock of pestilence occurred when the economic situation was depressed by very high production costs and intense foreign competition, the rise in salaries consequent upon the epidemic could aggravate existing problems. This must have been what happened in Florence as a result of the 1630 plague epidemic.

Another element which influenced the economic consequences of an epidemic was the size of the area affected. If the area was small, the gaps created by the plague could easily be filled by immigrants from neighbouring areas, with the consequent cancellation, or at least reduction, of any advantages obtained by the local labour force. If, on the other hand, the area affected was very large, the relative scarcity of labour compared to capital which ensued could not easily be eliminated or even substantially reduced in the short run and the only areas which would benefit from immigration from surrounding territories were the outlying areas.

The discussion does not end here, however. There were weighty institutional factors which had an overwhelming influence on the impact of a plague epidemic on the economy of the affected society. As we saw in the first chapter, Italy was at the forefront of Europe in matters of public health organisation during the fifteenth, sixteenth and seventeenth centuries. This had its positive aspects but also some negative ones, due above all to the mistaken medical theories which then prevailed. When a town or village was invaded by plague, the system of health boards throughout the whole of Northern Italy immediately sounded the alarm and went into action. The first step being to place the affected town or village under quarantine. This meant that all forms of communication and exchange were forbidden. The affected town or village thus found itself completely isolated, with consequent cessation of all traffic and exports and therefore the complete collapse of all commercial and manufacturing activity. When plague struck Busto Arsizio in 1630 a chronicler noted that the locally produced cotton cloth had been banned from every part of Italy 'just as the Devil is banned from Paradise'. During the 1657 pestilence the export of silk from Genoa dropped by 96 per cent. During the pestilence of 1630 in Florence the duties paid by the main Florentine trading companies to the firm that handled the mail also fell by 96 per cent, which indicates a corresponding reduction in commercial activity. These drastic contractions of trade obviously had a proportional effect on the general level of economic activity and on employment. In October 1575 Marcantonio Corsini, a representative of the city of Verona, whose cloth production was totally paralysed by the quarantine imposed on the city because of plague, travelled to Venice to obtain the suspension of the blockade. Corsini reported that many people had died of starvation because of unemployment and added that the unemployed could not hope for any help since they were imprisoned in a city under quarantine.

Typhus did not normally cause anything like the same degree of demographic ruin as the plague. The fatality rate of typhus in the absence of effective treatment was generally around 20 per cent; however, given the high incidence of the disease, the number of deaths could be high. In Florence between October 1620 and June 1621 under the pressure of a typhus epidemic the general mortality rate reached a level which, calculated on an annual basis, seems to have approached 60 per thousand, that is almost double the mortality rate in normal years.[3] In Castelfiorentino in 1627 typhus pushed the general mortality rate in the two months of August and September to a level equivalent to an annual rate of more than 300 per thousand (p. 65). In the view of Professor Del Panta, on the basis of available documents 'it is difficult to resolve the problem of a possible selectivity for age in petechial typhus [in the sixteenth and seventeenth centuries]'.[4]

Given its much lower fatality rate, typhus did not inspire the same degree of terror as the plague. A place which was overrun by a typhus epidemic was not placed under quarantine from other towns and villages and escaped the economic collapse which overtook places afflicted by plague.

Smallpox appears only once in the reports quoted above, at Campiglia in the spring of 1611 (pp. 43–4), and as usual it wreaked havoc among children: more than twenty children died in a month out of a population of a thousand, which, given the population structure of the time, presumably meant a population of about 300 children aged between 0 and 9 years. Obviously an epidemic which struck the youngest age groups selectively had, *ceteris paribus*, far more damaging economic consequences than an epidemic which affected different age groups equally.

One of the most striking facts in the reports quoted above is the prevalence of malaria in Tuscany outside the traditional malarial areas of the Maremmas. This is confirmed by various sources. L. Castelvetro wrote to G.B. Ferrari in 1552 that 'Pisa is not a place you should stay in after May if you value your life'.[5] G.B. Cartegni's 'Trattato de' Venti' (par. 3.3.) published in 1628 is a small book of little value but we read in it that 'the abundance of stagnant water renders the air [of Pisa] unhealthy in the summer and at the end of summer'.[6] In 1836 Dr Carlo Pucciardi, writing 'Della qualità dell'aria di Pisa' asserted that in Pisa from the Middle Ages on 'every year at the end of summer and in the early autumn months there were outbreaks of marsh fevers which left those they did not kill weak and full of the seeds of various sicknesses'.[7] According to Professor David Herlihy it was 'after 1250' that 'malaria worked its full havoc' in Pisa. At the end of the thirteenth century, still according to Professor Herlihy, 'every summer half of Pisa was infested'.[8]

Pisa was not an isolated case. Before drainage in 1591 the Val di Chiana was also infested with malaria, as were the Val di Nievole, and the valleys of the Paglia, the Orcia, the Era and the Elsa. The town of Luni was abandoned in the fifteenth century because of malaria.[9]

There is no lack of evidence nor of general information. What is lacking is a history of malaria which pinpoints accurately its geographical extent, the levels of and fluctuations in morbidity, and the possible cycles of recrudescence and remission.

Malaria is not only a great public health problem and a human tragedy: it also represents a huge economic problem. Malaria often does not kill, but it weakens its victims and severely undermines their productivity, acting as a determining factor in poverty and economic stagnation. Repeated attacks of malaria are generally responsible for the development in patients of 'malarial cachexy' which is characterised by emaciation, anaemia, extreme physical weakness and an abnormal psychological state characterised by inability to concentrate, loss of memory and a marked tendency to depression. What was the impact of malaria on the economic history of Tuscany over the centuries? And how do we explain the exuberant flowering of Tuscan culture, materially as well as artistically and intellectually, in an environment under siege from malaria? The question remains open.

Appendix

Ordinance of the Florence Health Officers, 4 May 1622

Since experience has often shown that contagions and sicknesses are caused mainly by the fact that in their houses or in the Towns, Villages and *Castelli* in which they live men are surrounded by dirt and by such quantities of filth that in well-ordered places there are statutes and orders which prohibit the keeping of rubbish in the streets, squares and other places; since this rubbish tends to give off smells and stenches which are so damaging to health; and since we are therefore continually careful that the inhabitants of this State should continue in the good state of health in which, by God's grace, they presently find themselves; desiring to take all necessary step to ensure that this is so; especially since we have been informed that in many places the good orders which we gave to this end are no longer observed: we order you immediately on our behalf and by public notice to command that in all the places under your jurisdiction everyone should remove and have removed from before their houses all the filth and rubbish which are to be found there, including manure and other things which can and do cause smells and stench; and that all that which is in the squares and other public places should be removed by the representatives of the Communities and be carried outside the Towns Villages and *Castelli* to places where they can do no harm; ensuring also that the greatest possible cleanliness be maintained in individual houses and that if there are full cesspits or other things that may cause damage by their smell, that they should be emptied and cleaned.

And furthermore make sure that care is taken around the sewers; and if there is water which is stagnant and can cause damage to health with the harmful vapours closed in as they are, that they should be given suitable outlets; and that the greatest care should be taken and that everything should be repaired in such a way that they are put right and cannot cause any harm to the inhabitants, for their health and preservation.

To this end you will call all the representatives of the Community and their Cancellieri to you and you will find out about their orders and statutes regarding this matter and you will take every care to see that they are observed; and where there are no orders and statutes on the subject, you will take such steps as you deem necessary and opportune, bearing in mind the nature of the place and its inhabitants, and any possible eventuality; and you will agree with these representatives and the Cancelliere to carry out these instructions and seeing as above that all filth and things harmful to health are removed; and to giving orders for the sewers, water and anything else that might cause harm; and you will send one of your Notaries to visit and ensure that everything is properly observed, with orders to him to note and observe whatever seems to need to be done in order to achieve the preceding effect by suggesting remedies; and you will inform this Magistracy of everything so that we may take the necessary steps according to what is needed; and you will ensure that everything is done quickly because after a month a competent person will be sent on a visit and if we find these orders of ours have not been carried out steps will be taken against the negligent.

Stay well.

4 May 1622

Notes

Introduction

1. F. Terranova, 'Le malattie degli italiani', in E. Sonnino (ed.), *Demografia e società in Italia*, Rome 1989, p.225.

Chapter 1 The Health Boards in Italy and Epidemiological Concepts

1. On the origin and development of the health magistracies in Northern Italy see C.M. Cipolla, *Public Health and the Medical Profession in the Renaissance*, Cambridge, 1973, ch. 1. The term 'health magistracies' is more appropriate than 'health boards' because these institutions had their own jurisdiction, their own courts, their own police force and their own prisons.
2. Cipolla, *Public Health*, pp.13–14.
3. See ibid., p.32ff.
4. Ibid., p.18ff. and C.M. Cipolla, *Fighting the Plague in Seventeenth-century Italy*, Madison, Wisconsin, 1981, pp.4–5.
5. Cipolla, *Fighting the Plague*, p.99ff.
6. G. Rosen 'Historical Trends and Future Prospects in Public Health', in G. McLachlan (ed.) *Medical History and Medical Care*, London and New York, 1971, pp.66–7, writes: 'It is indeed noteworthy that the programme of the sanitary reformers was to a large extent based on erroneous theories, and while they advocated appropriate solutions it was chiefly for the wrong reasons.'
7. C. Singer, *A Short History of Medicine*, Oxford, 1962, p.215.
8. Ibid.
9. A. Corbain, *Le miasme et la jonquille*, Paris, 1982.
10. P. Camporesi, Introduction to A. Corbain, *Storia sociale degli odori*, Milan, 1983.
11. In their furious aversion to the entire medieval heritage the eighteenth-century followers of the Enlightenment found fault even with the health magistracies' practice of carrying out inquiries and health inspections. Thus for example in 1770 Pietro Leopoldo d'Asburgo Lorena complained that 'the above-mentioned Health Magistracy spent money on purges for consumptives, the dispatch of doctors every time

there was a suspicion of disease of men or beasts in Tuscany'. See Pietro Leopoldo d'Asburgo Lorena, *Relazioni sul governo della Toscana*, ed. A. Silvestrini, Florence, 1977, pp.152–3. The criticism is both undeserved and senseless.

12. On community doctors in Tuscany in the first half of the seventeenth century, see Cipolla, *Public Health*, part II.

Chapter 2   'Miasmas, Filth and Rubbish'

1. ASF. Sanità, Negozi, b.139, c.687.
2. Ibid., cc. 49ss.
3. For Florence cf. C.M. Cipolla, *I pidocchi e il Granduca*, Bologna, 1979. The typhus epidemic broke out in Florence between September and October 1620, died down in the following summer but flared up again in the spring of 1622, lasting until the end of spring 1623.
4. ASF. Sanità, Negozi, b.139, c.523.
5. L. Del Panta, *Una traccia di storia demografica della Toscana nei secoli XVI–XVIII*, Florence, 1974, p.14. The 1622 census was the third of the population of Forence and the Florentine state. The two previous censuses were carried out in 1552 and 1562.
6. For all the above see ASF. Sanità, Negozi, b.135, c.153ff: report of Lorenzo Lucini, master mason, 15 September 1607.
7. ASF. Sanità, Negozi, b.136, c.701.
8. Ibid., b.135, c.868.
9. Ibid., b.139, c.808.
10. Ibid., b.135, c.672.
11. Ibid., c.689.
12. Ibid., b.139, c.526.
13. Ibid., c.596.
14. Ibid., c.530.
15. Ibid., c.639. 360 *scudi* were equivalent to 2520 lire. At the time a *libbra* (pound) of veal cost 6 *soldi*, a *libbra* of mutton 6 *soldi*, a *libbra* of goat meat 6 *soldi*, a *libbra* of salted meat 10 *soldi*, a *libbra* of lard 10 *soldi*.
16. ASF. Sanità, Negozi, b.139, c.639.
17. Ibid., c.444.
18. Ibid., b.135, c.153.
19. Ibid., c.231.
20. Ibid., b.136, c.43.
21. Ibid., b.135, c.153.
22. Ibid., b.136, c.449. In October 1631 an agreement was reached in Pontedera 'that in future it will be forbidden to keep the following items, subject to the following penalties, that is pigs, penalty 5 lire per pig, sheep, penalty 5 *soldi* each, quantities of liquid and solid manure and other filth, 7 lire per heap; anyone who throws excrement or urine or any other filth on to the streets 7 lire each, each time'. Cf. ASF. Sanità, Negozi, b.136, c.1292.
23. Ibid., c.1295.
24. ASF. Sanità, Copialettere, b.54, c.60v.
25. ASF. Sanità, Negozi, b.135, c.153.
26. Ibid., b.139, c.639.
27. Ibid., b.143, c.186.
28. Cipolla, *I pidocchi e il Granduca*, p.60.
29. ASF. Sanità, Negozi, b.135, c.153.
30. Ibid., c.961.
31. Ibid., b.142, c.597.
32. Ibid., b.139, c.526.
33. Ibid., c.530.

34. Ibid., c.577.
35. Ibid., b.136, c.701.
36. Ibid., b.143, c.177.
37. Ibid., b.142, c.595.
38. Ibid., b.135, c.899.
39. Ibid., b.139, c.530.
40. Ibid., c.560.
41. Ibid., c.577.
42. Ibid., b.135, c.153.
43. Ibid.
44. Ibid., b.138, c.35.
45. Ibid. b.142, c.534.
46. Ibid., b.137, c.327.
47. ASF. Sanità, Copialettere, b.54, c.94.
48. Pietro Leopoldo d'Asburgo Lorena, *Relazioni sul governo della Toscana*, ed. A. Silvestrini, Florence, 1977, vol.1, p.140.
49. ASF. Sanità, Negozi, b.135, c.153.
50. Ibid.
51. Ibid., b.136, c.173.
52. Ibid., b.139, c.601.
53. Ibid., c.672.
54. Ibid., b.140, c.1096.
55. Ibid., b.139, c.577.
56. Ibid., c.639.
57. Ibid., b.142, c.573.
58. ASF. Sanità, Decreti e Partiti 5, c.79v.

Chapter 3   Medical Reports and the Florentine Health Magistrates

1. C.M. Cipolla, *Public Health and the Medical Profession in the Renaissance*, Cambridge, 1973, p.124.
2. Ibid., p.118.
3. For example Francesco Bartolini, who was doctor in Peccioli in 1622, reappears in 1630 in Scarperia without an official post. Cipolla, *Public Health*, p.118.
4. It should be noted that the parish death registers include neither the age of the deceased nor the cause of death. Normally the doctors obtained this information from the parish priest, who relied on his own memory. Dr Bagnone makes this comment referring to his visit to Ponte Sacco (p. 39) when he writes: 'I had the number and names of the deceased from the parish priest who writes them in a book. I obtained information about the nature of the sickness from him, since he visited them many times, and from the local surgeon.'
5. For more details on the figures in the Vico parish register for 1609–10 see p.29.
6. C.M. Cipolla, 'The Bills of Mortality of Florence', *Population Studies*, 32.
7. Ludovico Pucci was born in Montepulciano and had studied in Pisa and Perugia 'per plures annos', graduating in philosophy and medicine in January 1572, Cf. L. Del Gratta: *Acta Academiae Pisanae*, Pisa, 1980, I, p.359.
8. ASF. Sanità, Negozi, b.135, c.386.
9. Dr Pucci's report can be found in ASF Sanità, Negozi, b.135, c.386.
10. ASF. Sanità, Copialettere, b.54, c.3v.
11. L. Del Gratta, *Acta*, pp.18 & 380.
12. Dr Pucci's report can be found in ASF. Sanità, Negozi, b.135, c.387ff.
13. Del Gratta, *Acta*, pp.18 & 380.
14. Dr Cartegni's report can be found in ASF. Sanità, Negozi, b.135, c.830.

15. Ibid., c.802.
16. F. aged 50, afflicted with a bad leg. She died after five days with catarrh falling from the throat, which could be seen from the tumour which appeared externally and from the difficulty she had in eating and drinking. And then it went down to her chest, which remained full of viscous humours, and since she was unable to cough them up she died of suffocation.

    M. aged 62, also died of catarrh in the throat and chest within four days, being unable to clear it. He had suffered greatly the previous year from being in prison for two months. Died 3 March.

    M. aged 35, weak by nature. Began to feel ill at two hours of the night with catarrh falling from his head and swelling his throat, making breathing and drinking difficult. Died 15 March.

    F. 31 years, she too with catarrh falling from the head to the throat and chest. Died after four days on 19 March.

17. M. died 3 February. More than 70 years old, after a long fever.

    M. died 4 February, having been sick for many years with fevers and other illnesses with catarrh descending to his chest.

    F. died 15 February of pleurisy after seven days.

    M. died 3 March: had been ill two or three years and died after catarrh descended to his chest.

18. M. aged 22 had been sick for 15 days with catarrh which descended first to the throat and then to the chest and has improved and will recover.

    M. aged 25 suffering from the same illness and will recover.

    M. aged 31, sick for eight days with the same catarrh in the throat and chest and greatly improved having coughed up most of the phlegm.

    M. suffering from asthma caused by the same catarrhs which descended to the chest several days ago and is not too ill.

19. M. died 14 March aged 28, with inflammation of the lungs and catarrh on the chest. Died after 17 days.

    M. died 18 March aged 30, with suffocating catarrh. Died after seven days.

    M. died 19 March aged 20, died of pleurisy after seven days.

    F. died 17 March aged 45, also died of catarrh in the throat and chest after three days.

    M. died 8 March of inflammation of the throat.

    M. from Monte Camoli, died after one day with catarrh in the throat and chest.

20. M. died 2 February, aged 30, had been badly afflicted with ulcerated legs and disorder of the spleen, died in one night with catarrh on the chest.

    M. died 4 February aged 44, after ten days of catarrh on the chest.

    F. died 8 February aged 35 after two days of catarrh on the chest; she had suffered from asthma some time before.

    F. died on 9 February aged 40, sickly: [died] after four days of swollen throat and catarrh on the chest.

    M. died 10 February aged 40, [died] in seven days of pleurisy.

    F. died 22 February aged 50, [died] in four days with catarrh and [had been] suffering from dropsy for many months.

    F. died 17 March, aged 25, [died] in eight days of post-partum fever.

    M. died 20 March, aged 53, died of dropsy.

    M. died 20 March, aged 70, [died] of catarrh in a few days. 'Most of the above received medical treatment.'

21. Dr Bagnone's reports can be found in ASF. Sanità, Negozi, b.135, cc.827, 871, 872, 873, 874, 875.

22.	sex	date of death	age	duration of illness (days)	remarks
	F	31.1	15	10	pneumonia & catarrh
	F	1.2	15	7	the same
	M	4.2	35	8	pleurisy, catarrh & death rattle
	M	5.2	44	7	the same
	F	9.2	40	7	catarrh on the chest
	F	18.2	55	8	the same
	F	24.2	22	5	the same
	M	27.2	–	3	convalescent of a long infirmity, died of catarrh which suffocated him
	M	10.3	55	5	the same

'Very few of these received treatment.'

23.	sex	date of death	age	duration of illness (days)
	M	29.1	32	7
	F	1.2	30	7
	M	14.2	63	5
	F	22.2	55	11
	M	26.2	22	4
	M	13.3	18	3
	M	15.3	30	7

24.	sex	date of death	age	duration of illness (days)	remarks
	F	1.2	24	7	catarrh on the chest having previously lost the power of speech
	F	3.2	65	few	with catarrh after a long illness
	M	10.2	10	8 hours	with catarrh on the throat and chest
	M	15.2		7	pleurisy or pneumonia
	M	20.2	10	7	pneumonia
	M	25.2	36	8	catarrh on the chest; had suffered for a long time
	F	28.2	28	7	pneumonia and catarrh on the chest
	F	2.3	51		long illness
	M	7.3	45	1	seriously ill before; believed to have died of apoplexy or catarrh on chest
	F	7.3	48	1	inflammation of the throat
	F	14.3	22	7	acute fever with delirium
	F	18.3	28	15	first erysipelas on the face then matter descending to the throat
	M	18.3	45	7	pneumonia
	M	19.3	63	7	pneumonia
	F	19.3	53	7	catarrh on the chest, was very sick before
	M	20.3		5 hours	catarrh on the chest, was very sick before
	M	20.3	35	15	after long sickness with catarrh which descended to the throat and chest

25. In January a male aged 25 'with an abcess on the chest'; in February a female aged 50 'with an abcess on one thigh'; in March an 80-year-old man 'died suddenly'.

26. Dr Bagnone's report can be found in ASF. Sanità, Negozi, b.135, cc.827, 871–5.

27. Ibid., c.826. As we shall see in the next section, in April 1611 Dr Ruschi was sent from Pisa to inspect Campiglia. The Pisan Magistrates, 'thinking that he would have to stay there some days', paid him 20 *scudi*. But Dr Ruschi finished the job very quickly and the Pisan Magistrates wrote that '[20 *scudi*] is perhaps too much for the short time he spent there, yet it does not seem right to ask for some of it back' (ASF.

Sanità, Negozi, b.136, c.23).

28. Ibid., b.135, c.858.

29. In the course of the sixteenth and seventeenth centuries, doctors' objections to the indiscriminate use of blood-letting had become increasingly frequent. Already in 1475 B. Reguardatus wrote in his 'Libellus de conservatione sanitatis' (in G. Deffenu, *Benedetto Riguardati*, Milan 1955, p.63) 'ad flobotamiam autem nunquam debemus esse prompti, nisi emergente necessitate aut impellent consuetudine, imo sanguinem qui est naturae tesaurus summopere custodire debemus'. In his *De contagione et contagiosis morbis*, book 3, ch.7 (Venice 1546) G. Fracastoro wrote on the subject of the 'Cura delle febbri veramente pestilenziali' ['The treatment of true pestilential fevers'] that 'in my opinion no phlebotomy should be practised in [the treatment of] these fevers'. In his *Avvertimenti sopra la peste* (Palermo, 1593) P. Parisi wrote that 'since there have been so many controversies and differing opinions between the ancients and moderns about this question of blood-letting . . . that so many problems have been created that it is impossible to know what to do'. During the plague of 1630 a doctor wrote to Cardinal Spada in Bologna: 'I must point out that purgatives and blood-letting are extremely dangerous in the plague and are rejected by the greatest doctors because the patient immediately loses strength'. On the other hand, Dr Francesco Cavazza, Reader in Medical Practice at the University of Bologna, practised blood-letting of patients 'usque ad animi deliquium' (A. Brighetti, *Bologna e la peste del 1630*, Bologna, 1968, pp.144 & 114). In his 'Relazione della carestia e della peste di Bergamo e suo territorio negli anni 1629 e 1630' (in *Miscellanea di storia Italiana* 6, 1865, p.436) M.A. Benoglio noted that 'among the doctors there were some, and in particular the distinguished Girolamo Pescina, Lazzaro Alghisi and Bartolomeo Locatelli who openly condemned any use of blood-letting'. In his book, *Il gran contagio di Verona* (Verona, 1631, pp.67–8), Dr F. Pona wrote that 'the emission of blood should be avoided. In this area of ancient surgical practices . . . the letting of blood was nothing less than a deviation of nature from its proper operation and functions.' A.F. Bertini wrote in his *La medicina difesa dalle calunnie degli uomini volgari e dalle opposizioni dei dotti* (Lucca, 1699, p.32): 'I know that in Naples it was formerly the practice to do a great deal of blood-letting and in particular for all kinds of inflammation and almost all fevers, whereas today none or very little blood-letting is done and most doctors abhor the practice.'

30. On Cartegni's statement about the number of deaths in Vico see above p.29.

31. ASF. Sanità, Negozi, b.136, c.17.

32. On 24 April the Capitano of Campiglia wrote in a letter to the Grand-Duke: 'I showed Signor Cesare [Ruschi] the book of those buried who number sixty: forty adults and twenty children, some of whom died of smallpox and other things' (ASF. Sanità, Negozi, b.136, c.18).

33. To be precise, 887 inhabitants in 1552 and 296 in 1632 after the plague epidemic.

34. Dr Ruschi's report can be found in ASF. Sanità, Negozi, b.136, c.19.

35. R. del Gratta, *Libra matricularum Studii Pisani*, Pisa, 1983, p.22 and Del Gratta, *Acta Gradum*, p.392.

36. ASF. Sanità, Negozi, b.136, c.588.

37. Ibid.

38. ASF. Sanità, Copialettere, b.54, c.43.

39. ASF. Sanità, Negozi, b.136, c.588.

40. Ibid., c.590.

41. ASF. Sanità, Copialettere, b.54, c.43.

42. Dr Ruschi's report can be found in ASF. Sanità, Negozi, b.136, c.607.

43. Ibid., c.610.

44. Ibid., c.759.

45. Ibid., c.1049.

46. ASF. Sanità, Copialettere, b.54, c.53.

47. ASF. Sanità, Negozi, b.136, c.1075.
48. Ibid., c.1160.
49. C.M. Cipolla, *Chi ruppe i rastelli a Montelupo?*, Bologna, 1977, p.25, n.2.
50. ASF. Sanità, Negozi, b.136, c.1081.
51. Ibid., cc.1080ff.
52. The register is preserved in the Archive of the Curia Vescovile in Florence.
53. It should be remembered that not all deaths were necessarily due to malaria.
54. C.M. Cipolla, *Fighting the Plague in Seventeenth-century Italy*, Madison, Wisconsin, 1981, p.40.
55. Dr Collodi's report can be found in ASF. Sanità, Negozi, b.137, c.291.
56. On the spread of typhus in the Marche and Romagna in the early 1620s see Cipolla and Monori, *Le Marche nell' epidemia di tifo petecchiale del 1662*, now in press.
57. C.M. Cipolla, *I pidocchi e il Granduca*, Bologna, 1979, pp.31–2.
58. Ibid., pp.33–5.
59. Ibid., chs. 2, 3 & 4.
60. ASF. Sanità, Negozi, b.138, cc.1136 & 1141; b.139, cc.4, 34, 75.
61. ASF. Sanità, Negozi, b.138, c.1137.
62. Dr Bargellini's report can be found ibid., c.1138.
63. Ibid., b.139, c.447.
64. Ibid., b.138, c.477.
65. Cf. Cipolla, *Public Health*, pp.76, 100–1, 113–4, 119.
66. L. Magalotti, *Lettere familiari*, Venice, 1719, part I, Letter XIII, p.202.
67. ASF. Sanità, Negozi, b.139, c.446. The following monthly mortality figures were provided by the Capitano:

May 1621	37
June	35
July	28
August	34
September	24
October	33
November	29
December	24
January 1622	31
February	33
March	36
April (to the 19th)	36

68. ASF. Sanità, Negozi, b.139, c.474.
69. Ibid., c.475.
70. Ibid., c.444.
71. Ibid., c.460.
72. Ibid., c.477.
73. Ibid., b.140, c.87.
74. Ibid., b.142, cc.569ff, 630ff.
75. Ibid., c.537.
76. Ibid., c.572.
77. The register is preserved in the Archive of the Curia Arcivescovile in Florence.
78. ASF. Sanità, Negozi, b.142, c.588.

Chapter 4 Doctors, Diseases and the People

1. C.M. Cipolla, *I pidocchi e il Granduca*, Bologna, 1979, p.72.
2. ASF. Sanità, Negozi, b.140, cc.222, 244.
3. Douglas Bennet Mandell, *Principles and Practice of Infectious Disease*, New York, 1986, p.1518.

4. Alessandra Macinghi negli Strozzi, *Lettere di una gentildonna fiorentina del secolo XV ai figliuoli esuli*, ed. C. Guasti, Florence, 1877, p.177, letter 17, 6 September 1459.
5. C.M. Cipolla, *Fighting the Plague in Seventeenth-century Italy*, Madison, Wisconsin, 1981, p.40.
6. E.D. Kilbourne, *Influenza*, New York, 1987, p.14.
7. ASF. Sanità, Negozi, b.139, c.48.
8. Ibid., b.140, c.87.
9. From the death register of Vico Pisano 1609–10 (kept in the Archive of the Curia Arcivescovile in Pisa) we obtain the following list of deaths:

		adults	'children'	total
1609	June	2	–	2
	July	4	–	4
	August	1	2	3
	September	5	5	10
	October	1	1	2
	November	3	–	3
	December	3	1	4
1610	January	1	4	5
	February	1	–	1
	March	2	1	3
	April	13	4	17

10. C.M. Cipolla, *Public Health and the Medical Profession in the Renaissance*, Cambridge, 1973, p.114.

Chapter 5   Conclusion

1. M.D. Grmek, 'Metodi nuovi nello studio delle malattie antiche', *Scienza e tecnica*, 75, Milan, 1975, p.75.
2. T. Thompson, *Annals of Influenza or Epidemic Catarrhal Fever in Great Britain from 1510 to 1837*, London, 1852, p.11.
3. C.M. Cipolla, *I pidocchi e il Granduca*, Bologna, 1979, pp.89ff.
4. L. Del Panta, *Le epidemie nella storia demografica italiana*, Turin, 1980, p.56.
5. *Alcune lettere di illustri italiani*, Modena, 1827, p.16.
6. G.B. Cartegni, *Trattato de' venti in quanto si appartiene al medico e del sito della città di Pisa*, Pisa, 1628, p.51. In the manuscript report on Marciana, Cascina and Pontedera sent to the Florentine Magistracy in 1610 (p.35ff), Dr Cartegni writes: 'This city of Pisa is located among many stretches of stagnant water and marshes which are often the cause of many serious illnesses at the end of summer, and especially when it is hotter than normal; this is because the water partly dries up around the edges and the mud and other matter putrefy together with the smaller quantity of water which remains; and very harmful vapours rise up from this putridity and corruption and are then carried by the wind to this part of the country and infest the bodies and bring many harmful sicknesses.' The aetiology of malaria was therefore explained by the 'putrefaction' of the edges of the pools caused by the lowering of the level of the stagnant water.
7. C. Pucciardi, *Della qualità dell'aria pisana. Dissertazione istorico-medica*, Pisa, 1836, p.13.
8. D. Herlihy, *Pisa in the Early Renaissance*, New Haven, 1958, p.49.
9. A. D'Ancona (ed.), *L'Italia alla fine del secolo XVI. Le memorie di viaggio di Montaigne*, Città di Castello, 1895, p.539, n.1.

Glossary

The translation of technical medical expressions of the seventeenth century presents often unsolvable problems. In many instances it is difficult, if not impossible, to interpret what contemporary doctors said or meant: technical language had not yet been standardised. To compound the difficulty, some terms were spelled differently by different doctors, such as *scherantia*, *scherentia* or *schiantia*, meaning 'inflammation of the throat'. This glossary seeks to explain medical – and political – terms which have no exact equivalent in twentieth-century English usage. It also identifies some English usages which are rare or antiquated.

Accidente
a bad symptom which occurs during an illness

Angina
inflammation of the throat which causes difficulty in breathing and swallowing

Bezoar
a hard stone obtained from the stomach or intestines of animals, and believed to be an antidote to poison

Cacochymy, -chymic
a rare term denoting an unhealthy state of the fluids and 'humours' of the body

Cancelliere
a chancellor

Castello
a Tuscan walled settlement, more than a village but less than a city

Capitano di Giustitia
a representative of the Grand-Duke, whose area of jurisdiction was the *Capitanato*

Commissario
a commissioner

Contadini
peasants who worked on the land

Electuary
a mixture of medicine with sugar, syrup or honey

Exanthema, -mata
a medical term, meaning an efflorescence, rash or skin eruption, in this case associated with typhus

Jewel alkermes
a medical confection of which the Kermes, or Scarlet Grain insect, was an ingredient

Juleb
a liquid prepared from sweetened boiled fruit

Lazaretto
a hospital for the poor and the sick, especially lepers and, in this case, victims of plague

Mal di punta
equivalent of a 'stitch'

Petechia (pl. *petechiae*)
hemorragic suffusions caused by the toxins of the rickettsie on the endothelial cells of the capillaries

Podestà (pl. *Podestà*)
a government official and representative of the Florentine Grand-Duchy

Provveditore (pl. *Provveditori*) *di sanità*
a commissioner of public health

Scherantia/schiranzie
a popular word for angina, spelled with many variants

Surgeon
a medical officer of low rank and status, distinct from physicians
who had a university training and hence high rank and status

Vesicant
a substance used medicinally to raise blisters on the skin

Vicario (pl. *vicari*)
a government official and representative of the Florentine
Grand-Duchy

Index